©2014 by HotFlashHell.com
Photography © 2014 by Wagoner Photography, Inc. and others

All rights reserved. No part of this book may be reproduced or transmitted in any form
(except for brief excerpts for the express purpose of review) without the written permission of the publisher.
This includes, but is not limited to, mechanical reproduction, electronic transmission, photocopying, and/or image insertion in email.
Requests for permission can be submitted to www.HotFlashHell.com.

Our thanks to the many friends and family members who helped make this book a reality.

The characters portrayed in this book are fictitious.
Any similarities to real persons, living or dead, are coincidental and not intended by the creators.

{ The only way a man could truly understand menopause would be if he were beaten senseless and set on fire. }

Until there's a safe, legal way to do that,
"Menopause It's Time Guys Got It" is the next best thing.

The symptoms on the following pages are real.

We (the menopausal authors) are treating these symptoms
with humor—because if we didn't laugh, we'd cry.

You (the non-menopausal male) should treat them more seriously—
because the menopausal women in your life
may be armed.

{ It's official.
You're married to
the hottest woman
on the planet. }

HOT FLASHES

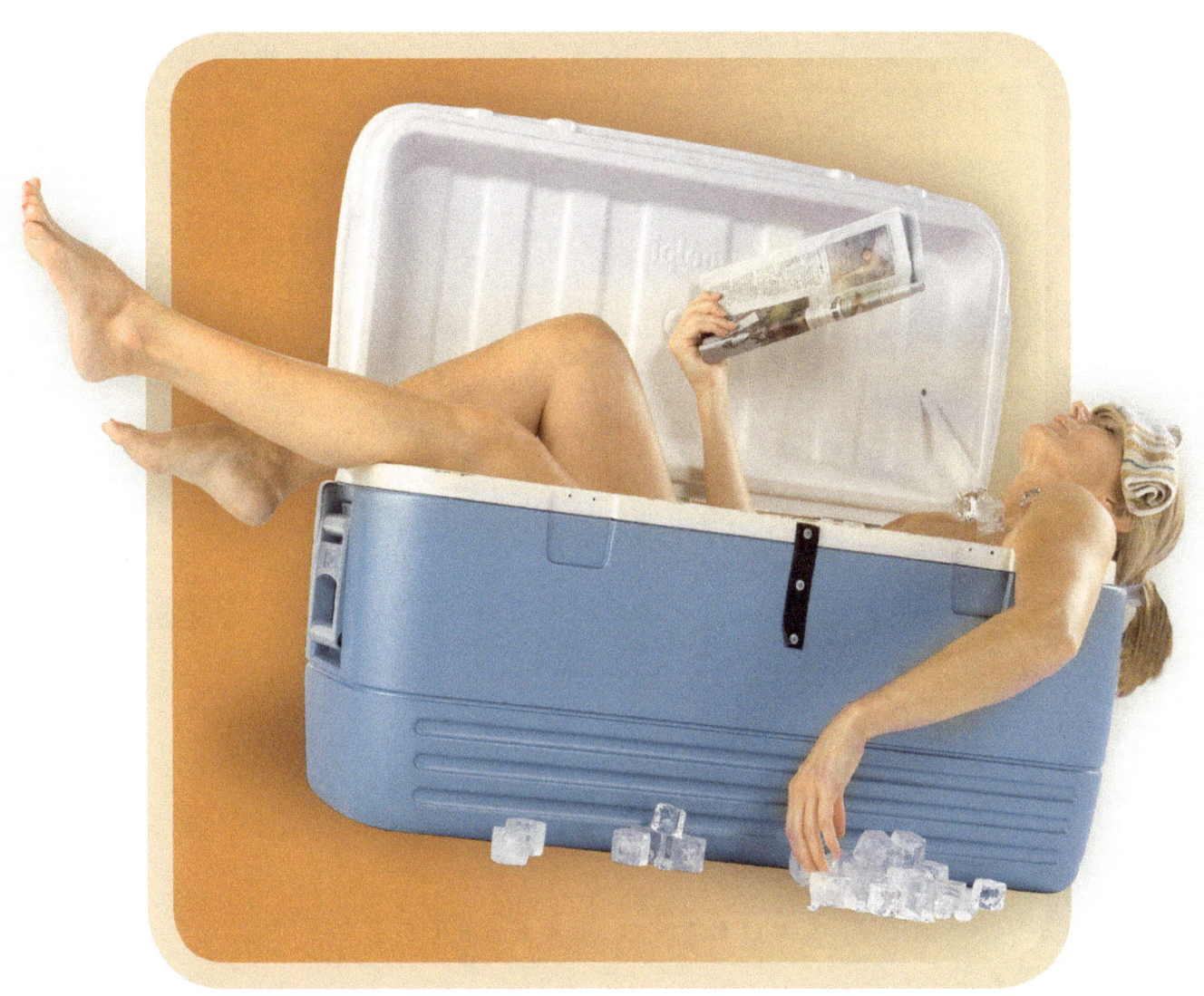

{ I can tie 'em in a knot.
I can tie 'em in a bow. }

SAGGING BREASTS

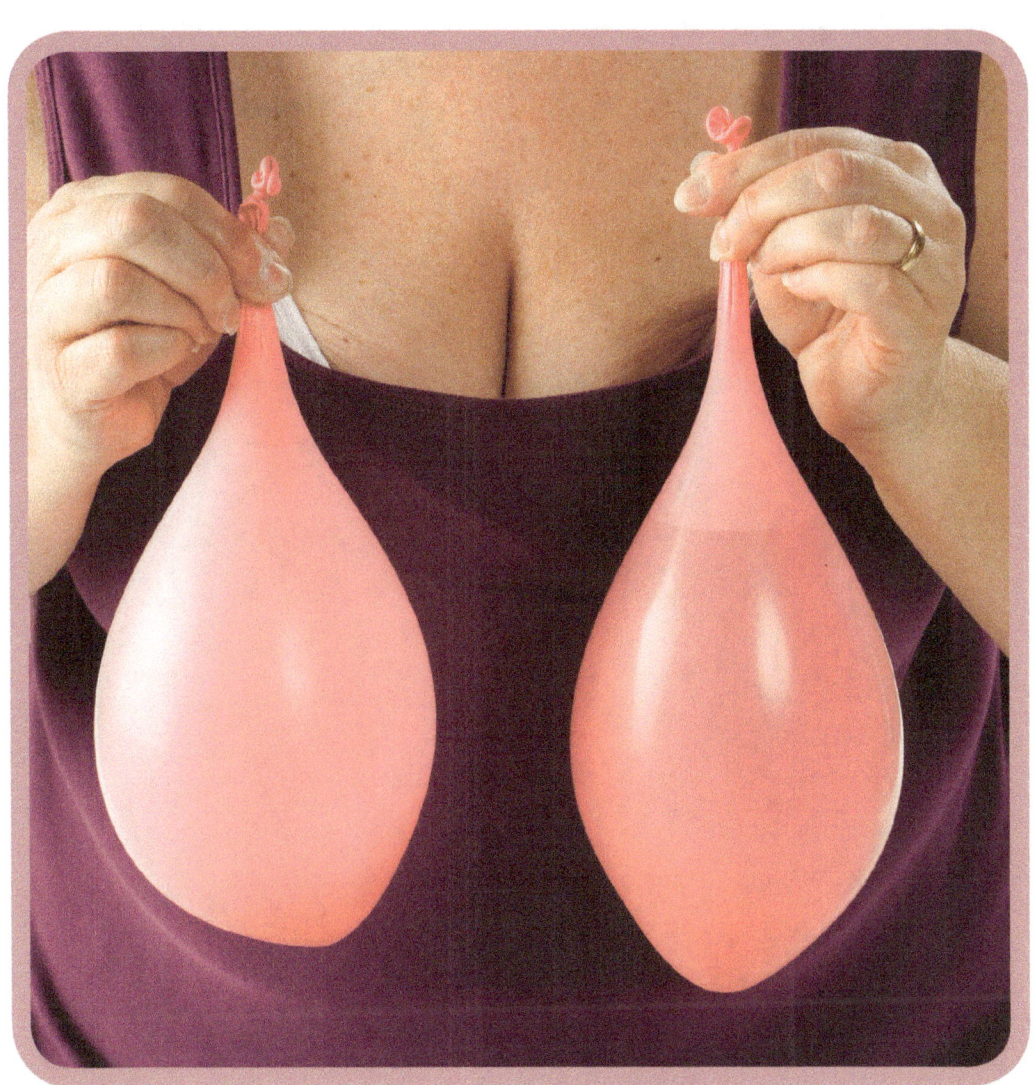

{ Lately,
you're more annoying
than Rusty. }

REDUCED LIBIDO

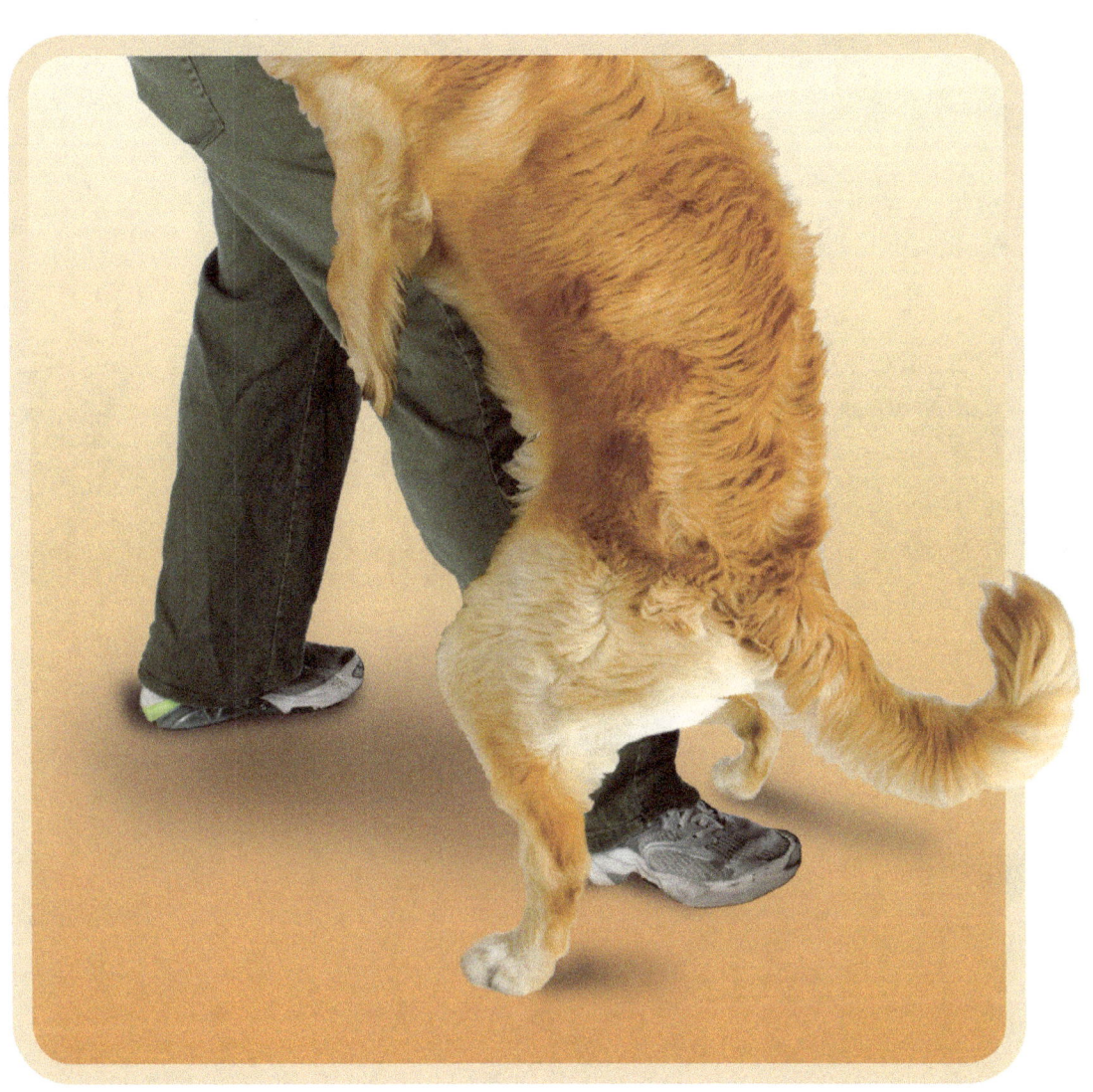

{ Not only do I
lie awake all night.
I lie awake
and look at this. }

INSOMNIA

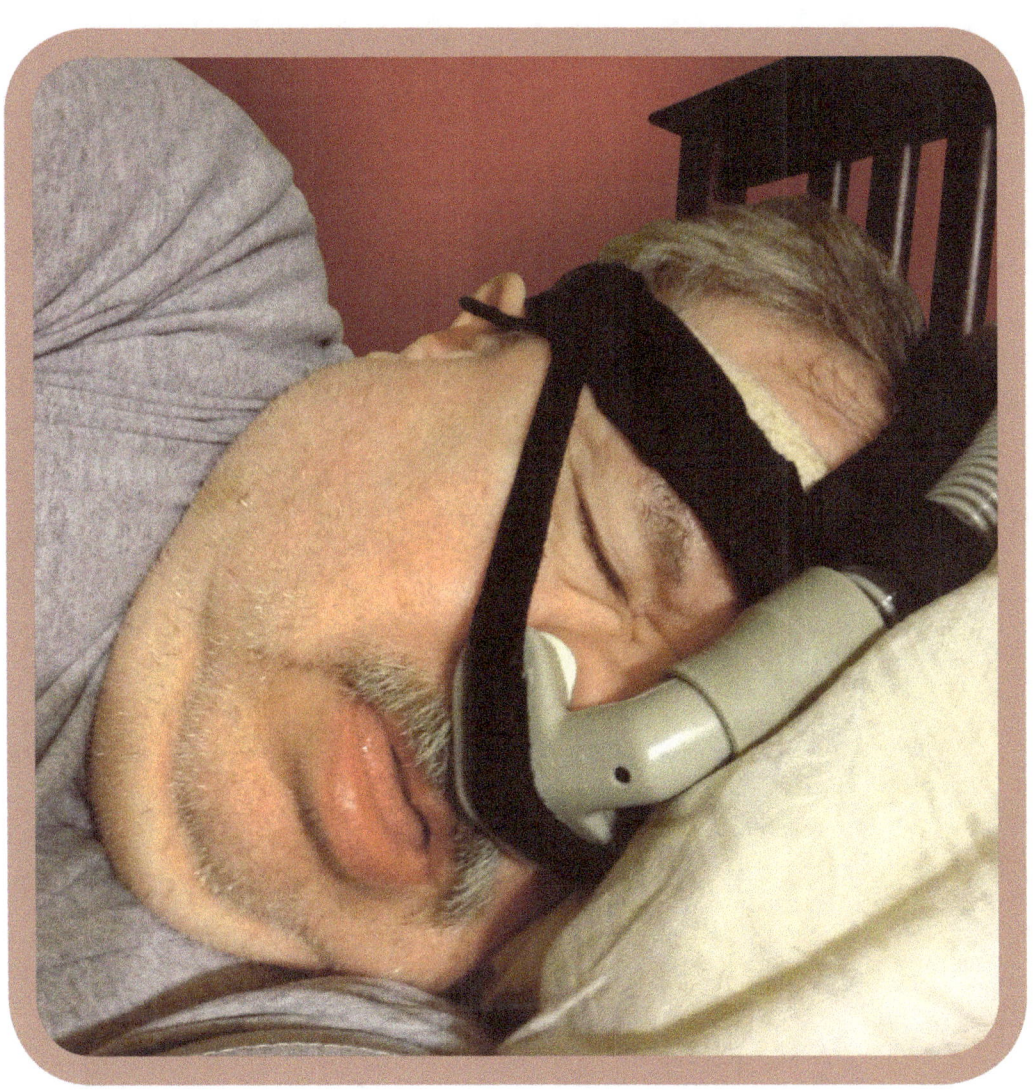

{ I'm so bloated,
you could rope my ankle
and put me in the
Thanksgiving parade. }

BLOATING

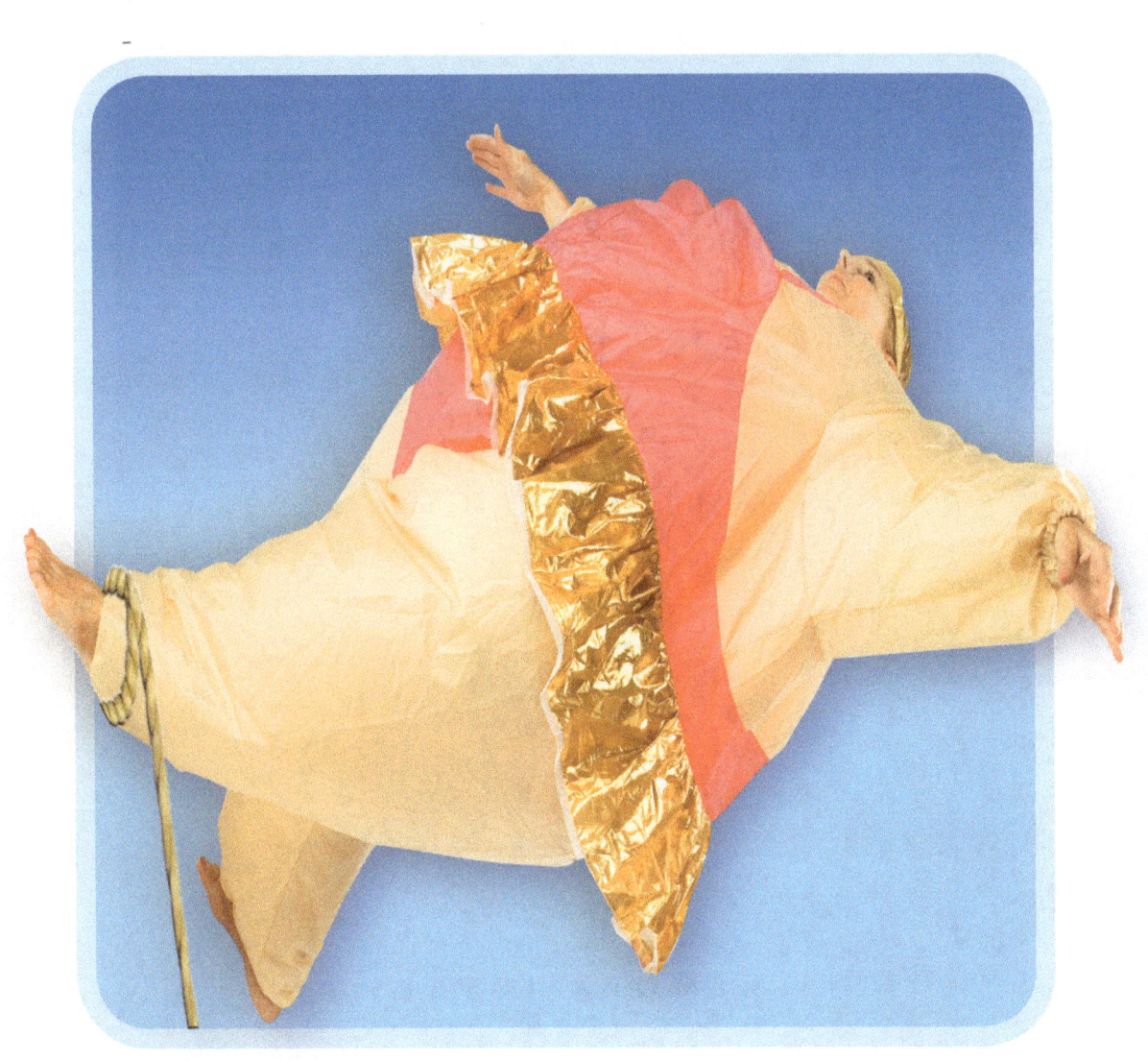

{ I leave myself notes
and wonder
who they're from. }

MEMORY LAPSES

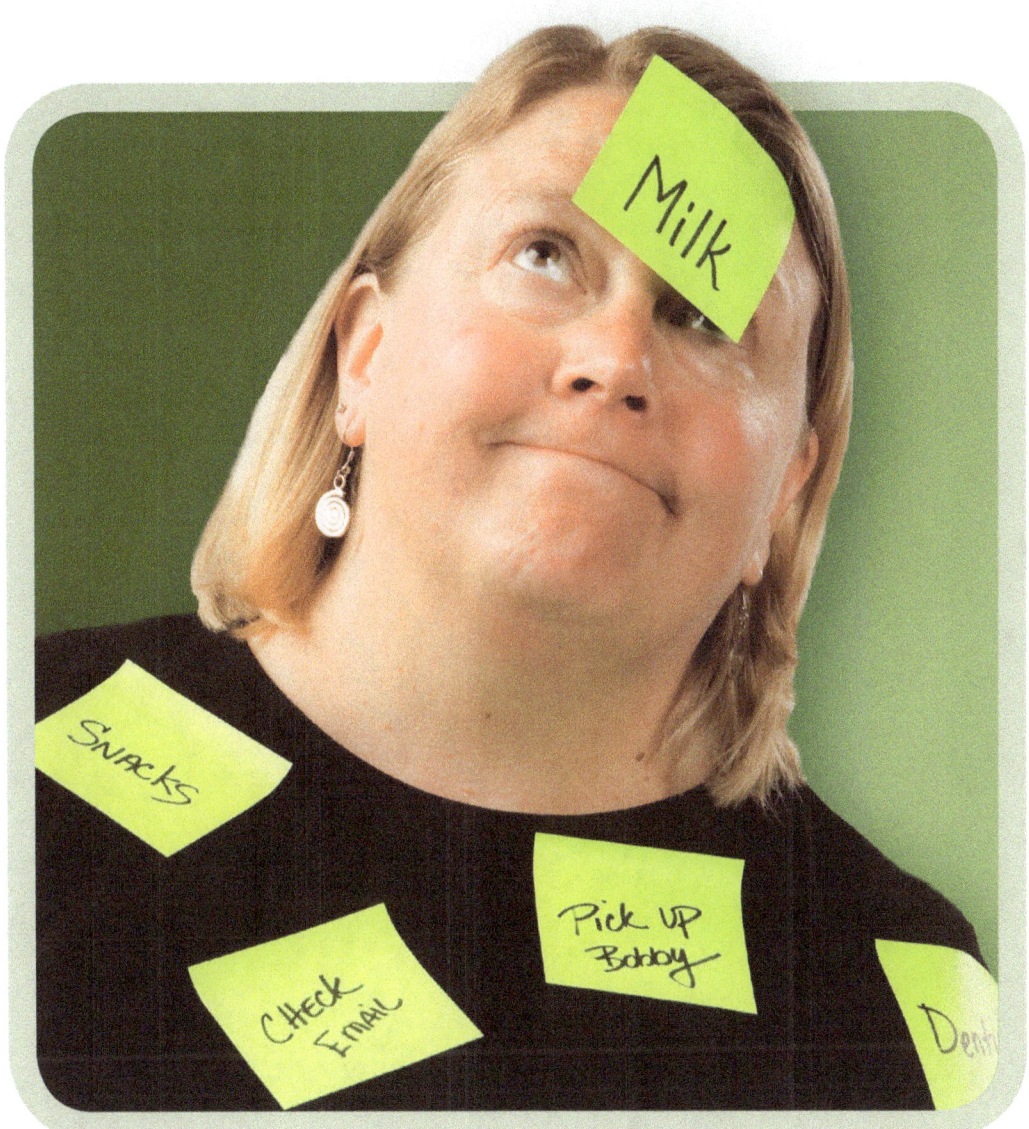

{ Do these hormones make my butt look big? }

WEIGHT GAIN

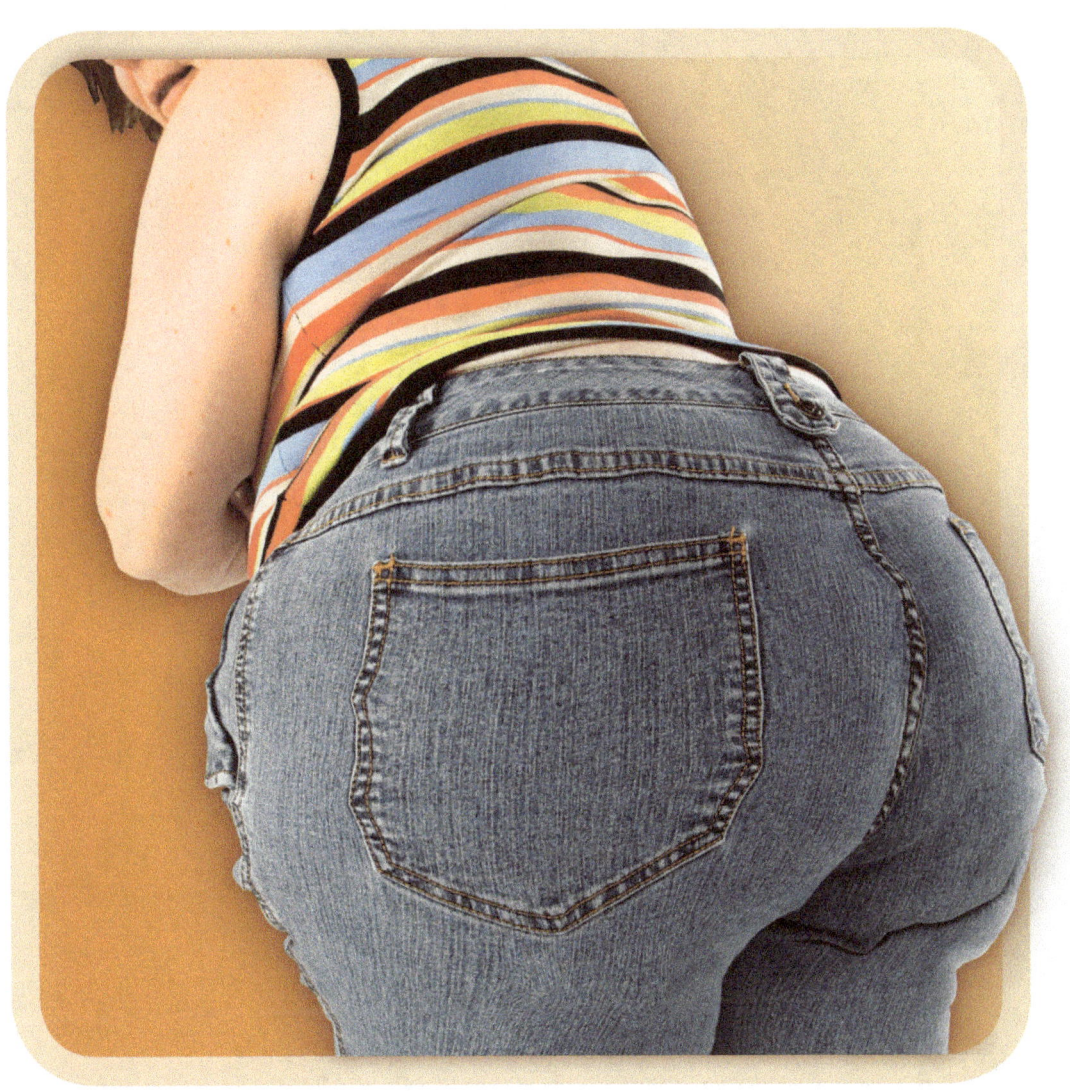

{ For years
you've tried to get me
all sweaty in bed.
Now that I am,
don't complain. }

NIGHT SWEATS

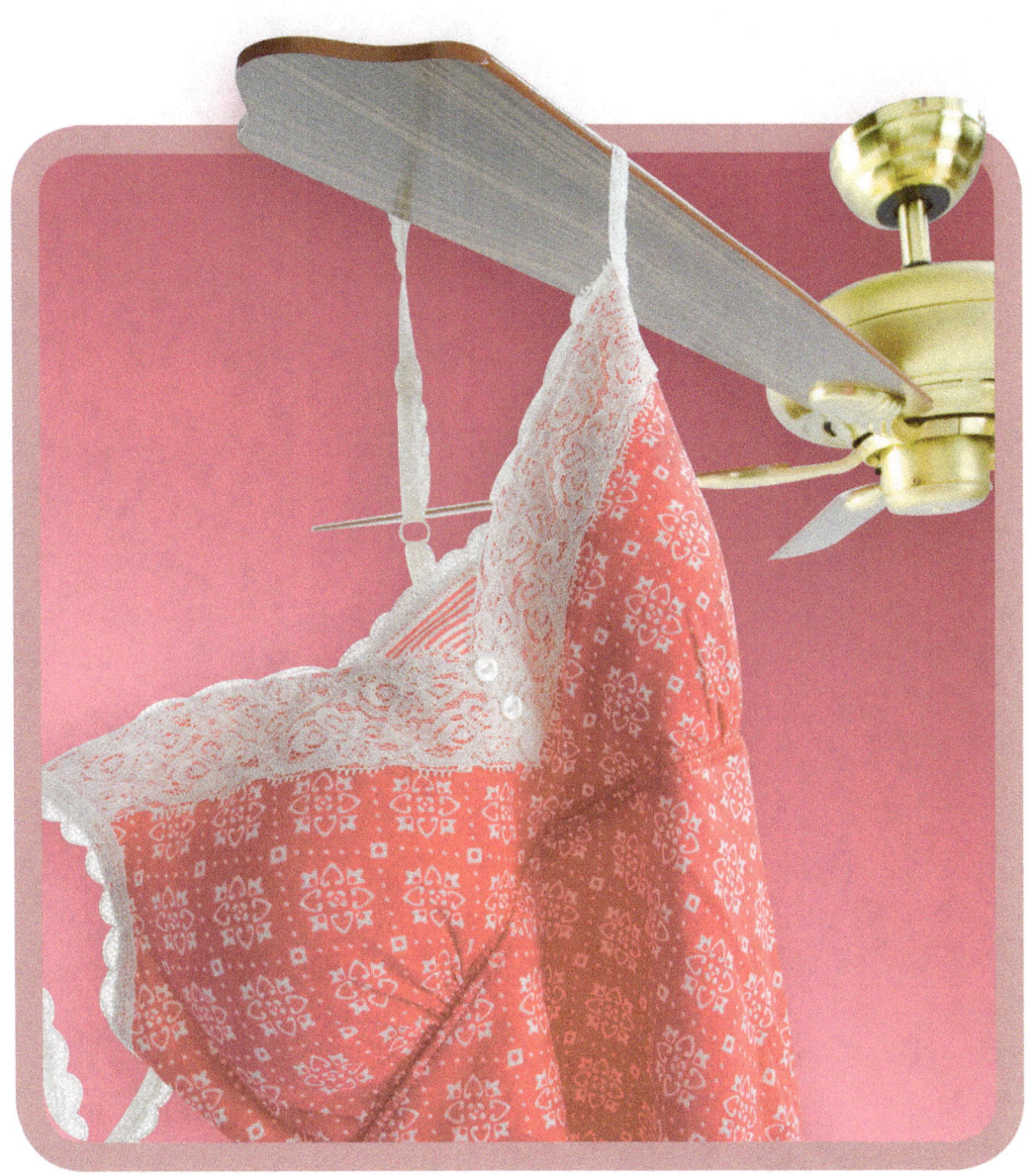

{ My brain chemicals are so unbalanced, I can't make rational decisions. What's your excuse? }

CONFUSION

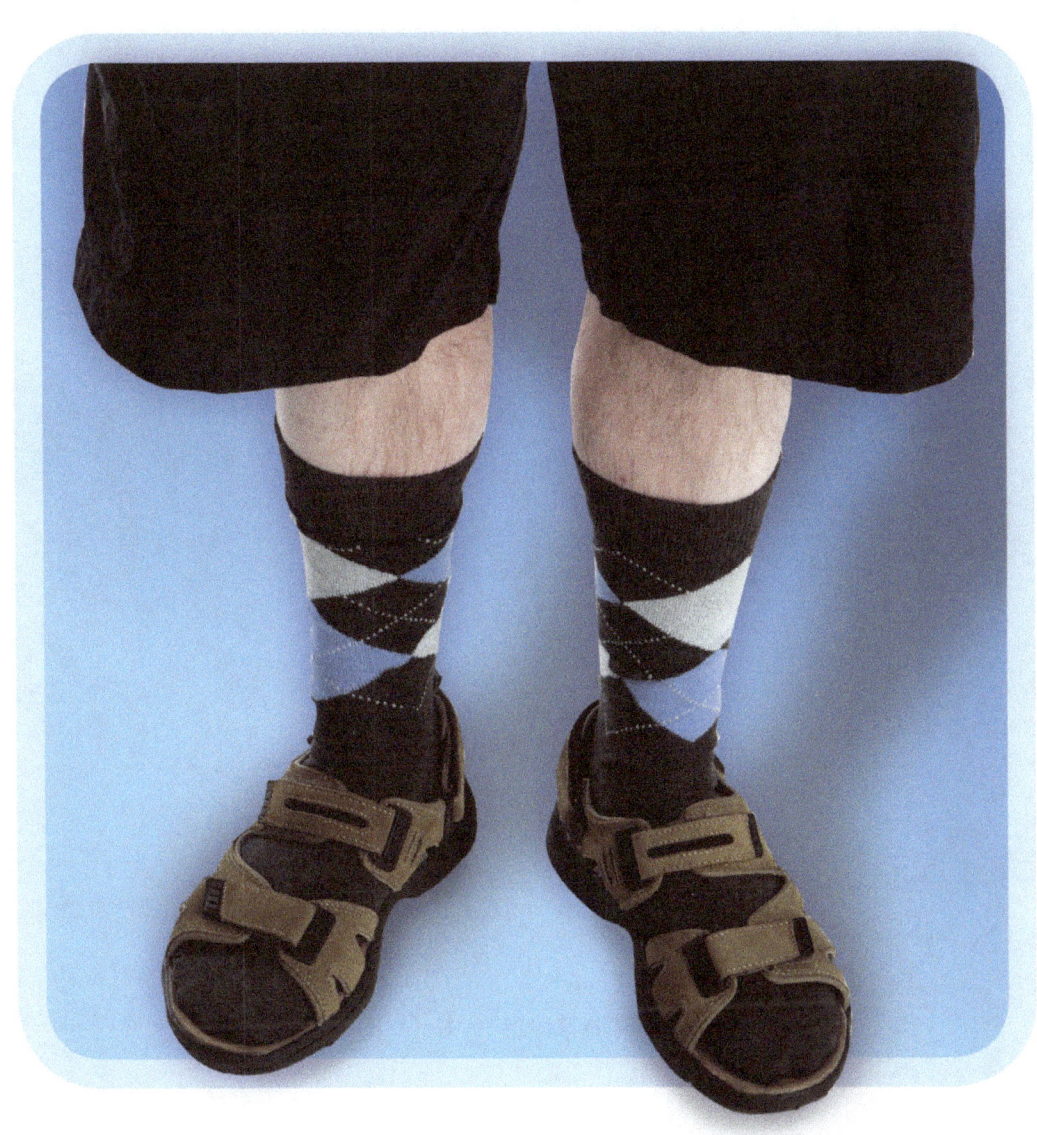

{ The part of
my body you like best
has shriveled up
and stuck to itself. }

VAGINAL ATROPHY

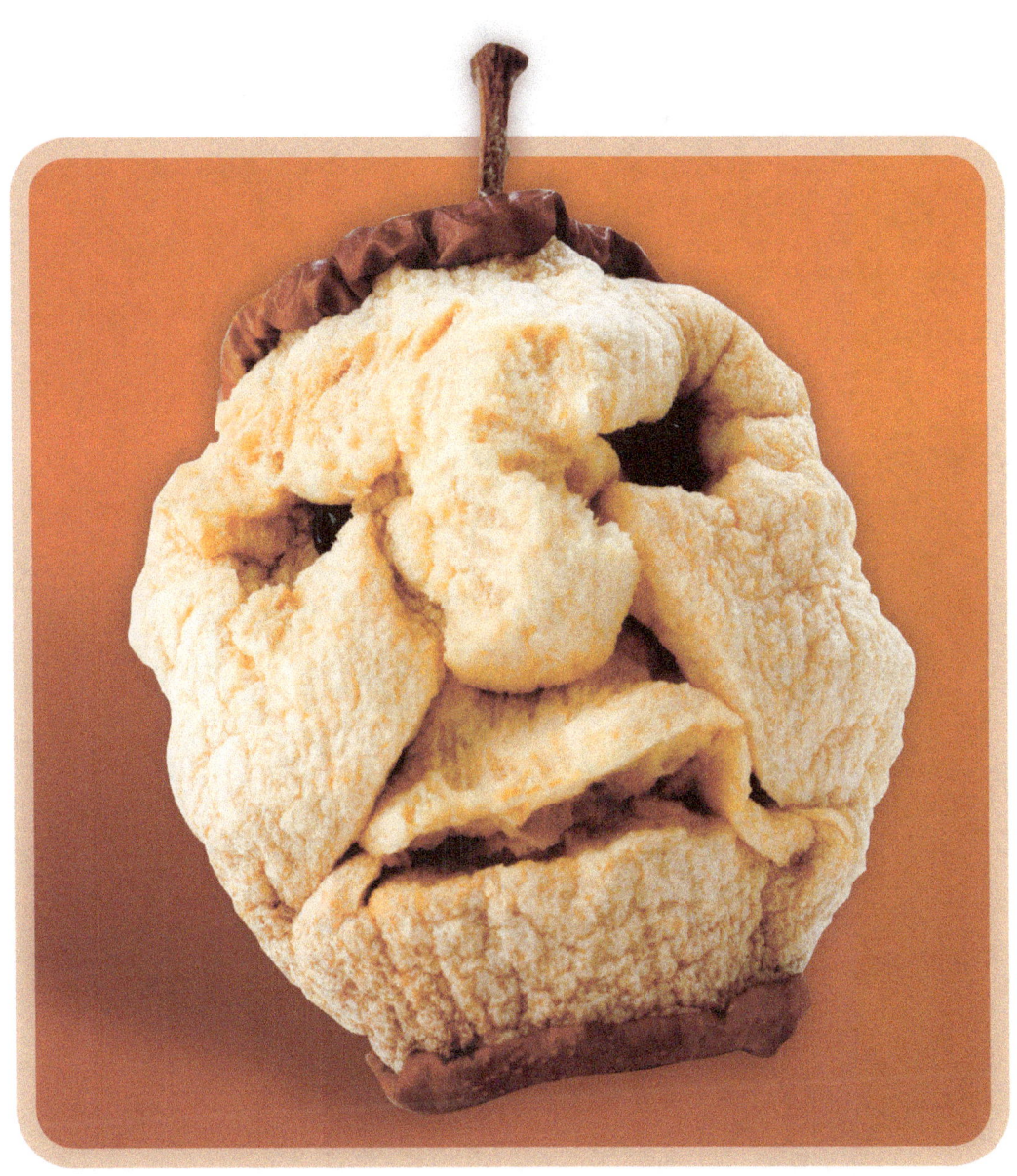

{ The zapping
under my skin could run
an 8-cylinder engine. }

ELECTRIC SHOCKS

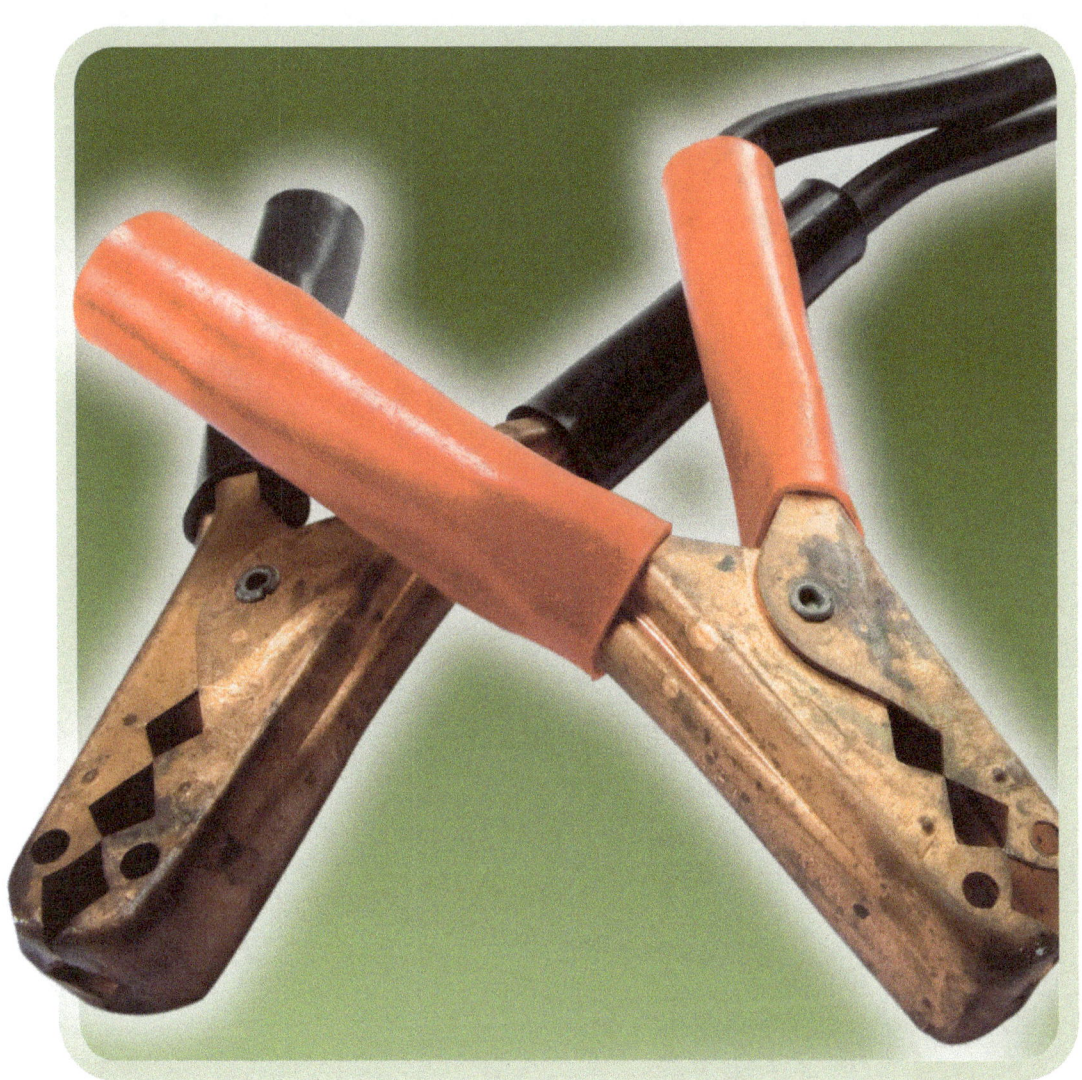

{ Shorts season is officially over. Forever. }

VARICOSE VEINS

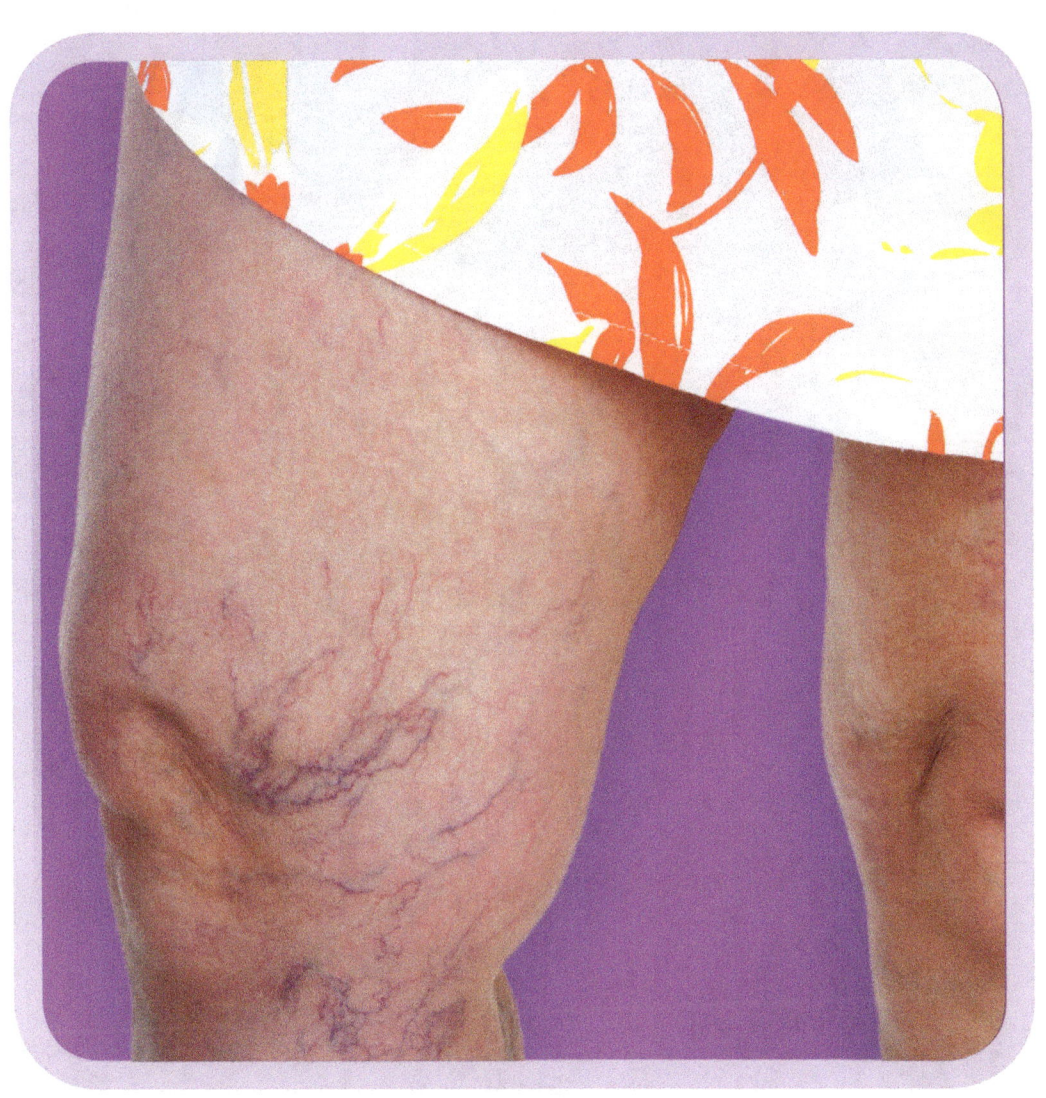

{ My period shows up
at odd times
for unknown durations.
Just like your mother. }

IRREGULAR MENSTRUATION

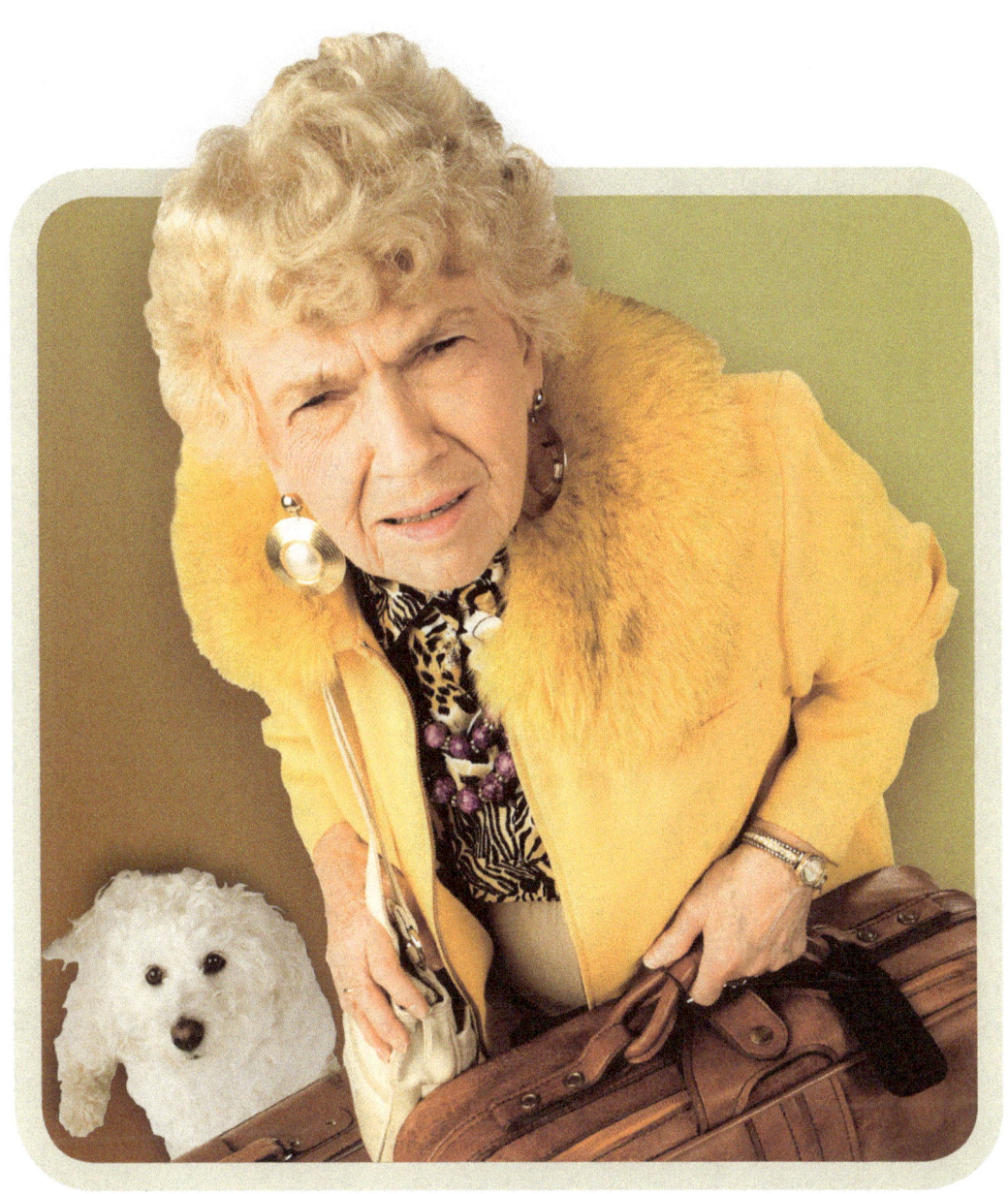

{ My hair's not falling out.
It's migrating to other parts
of my head. }

HAIR LOSS (& GAIN)

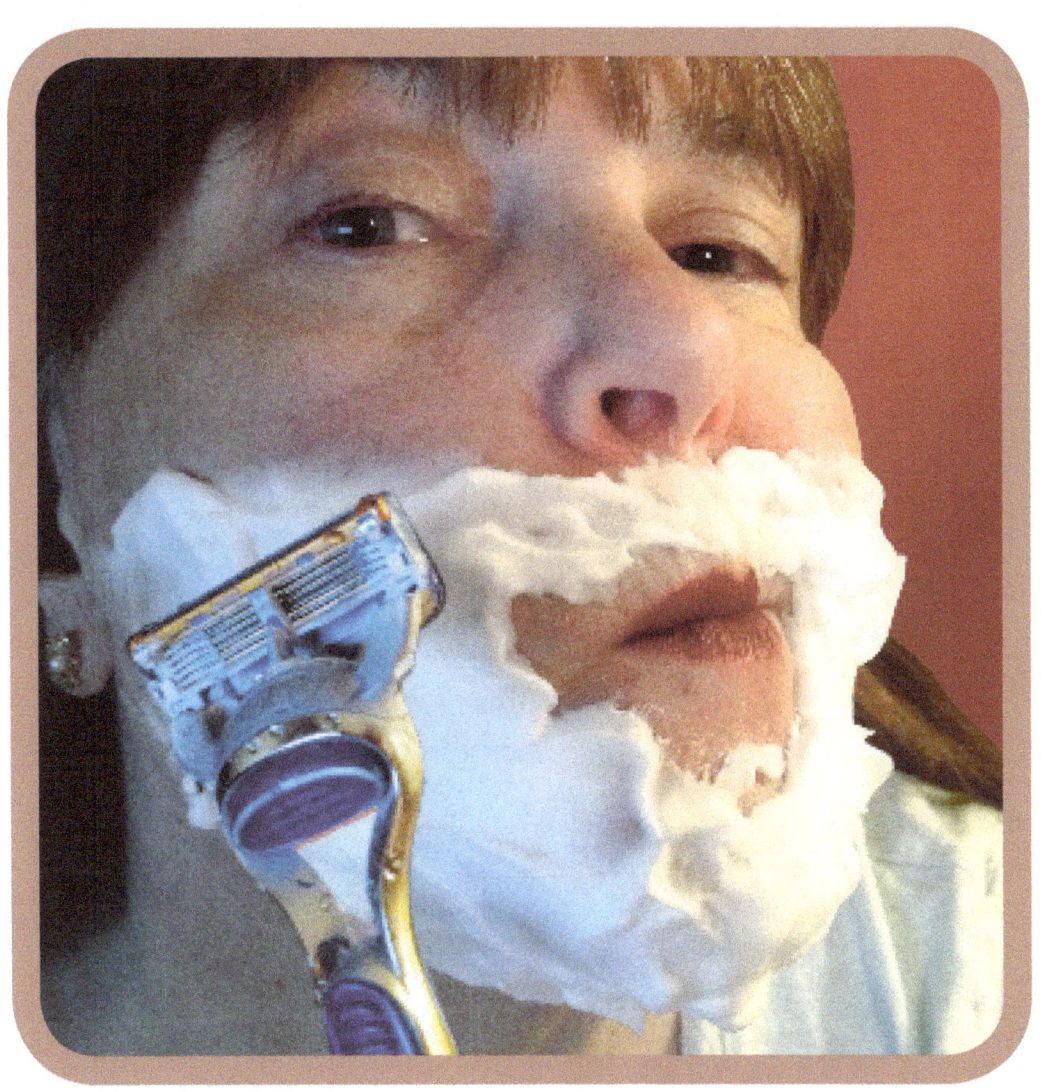

{ Nature is
getting back at me
for all the times I *said*
I had a headache. }

MIGRAINES

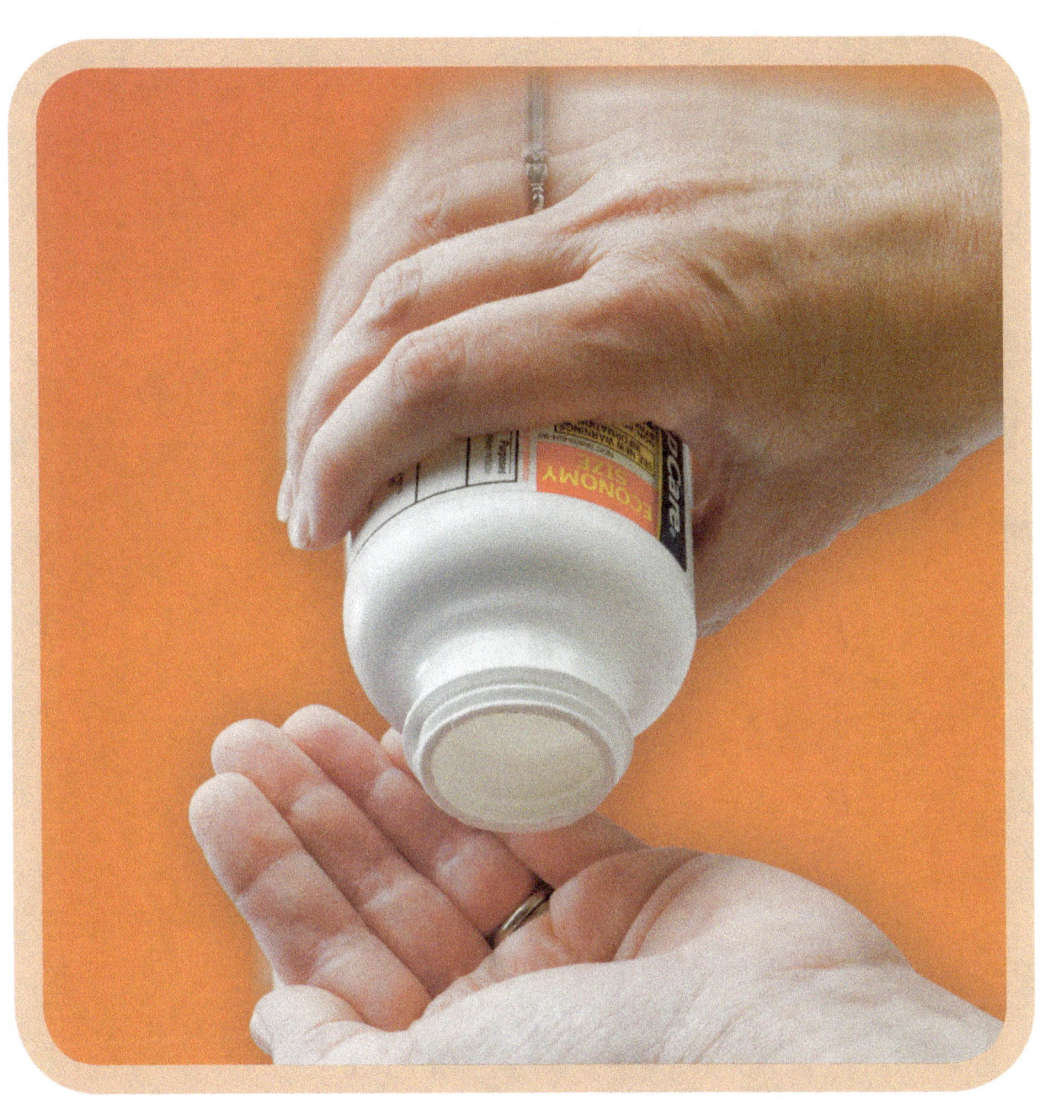

{ I can
barely focus anymore.
Perhaps,
that's a *good* thing. }

DIFFICULTY CONCENTRATING

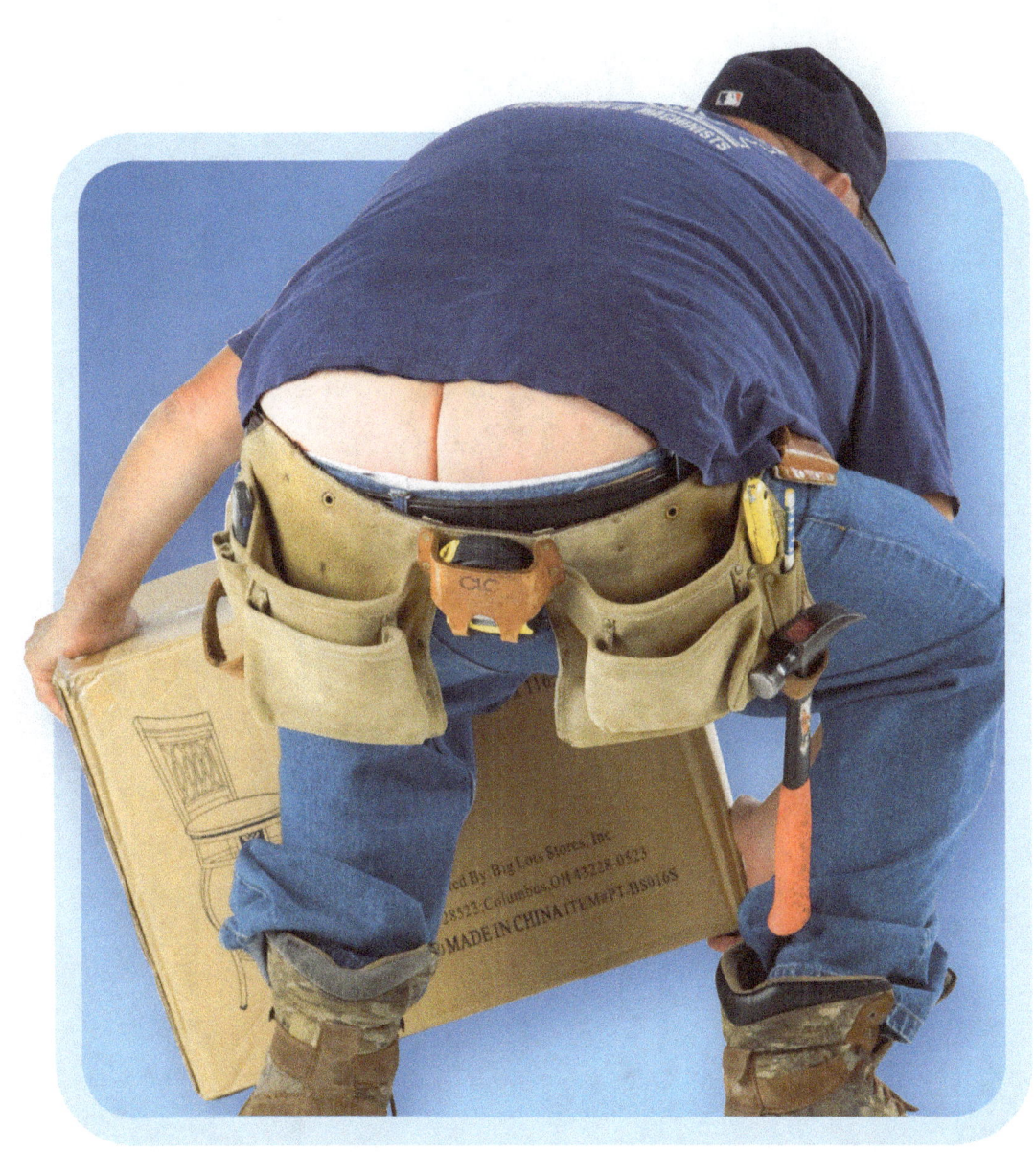

{ I've been reduced to taking pills made out of horse pee. }

HORMONE IMBALANCE

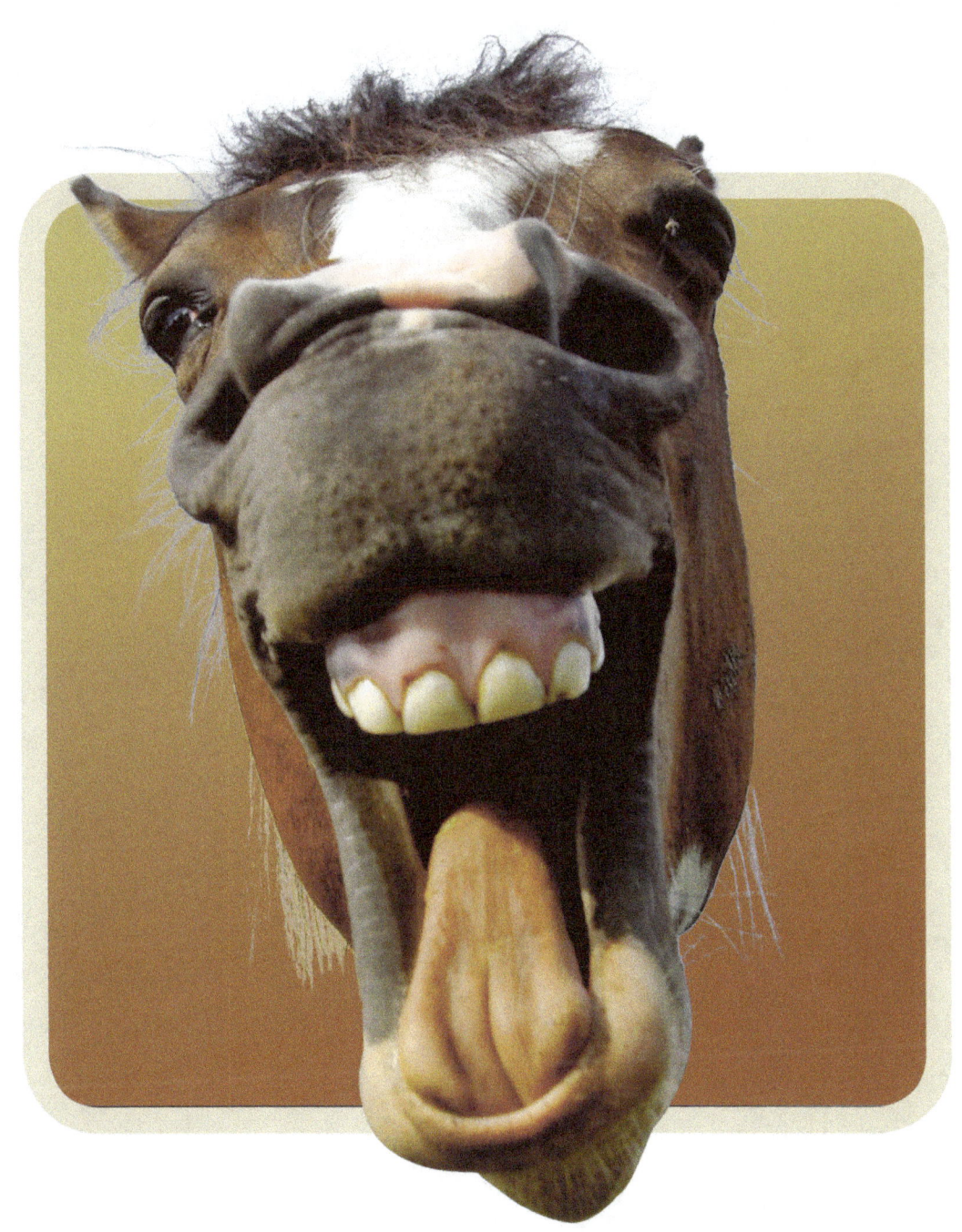

{ My mood ring
goes from blue to black
in 10 seconds flat. }

MOOD SWINGS

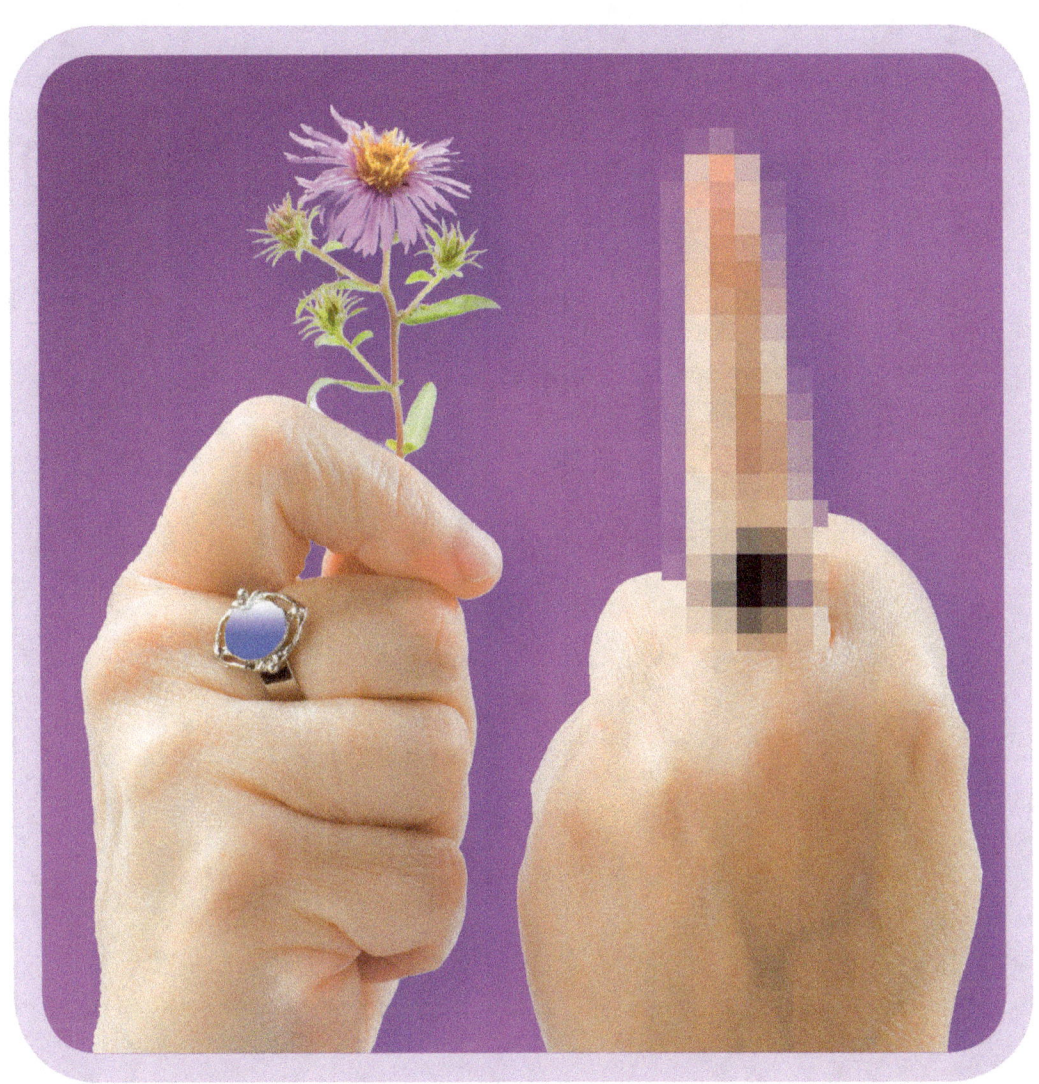

{ It's not just heating and cooling— now I have plumbing issues, too. }

DIGESTIVE PROBLEMS

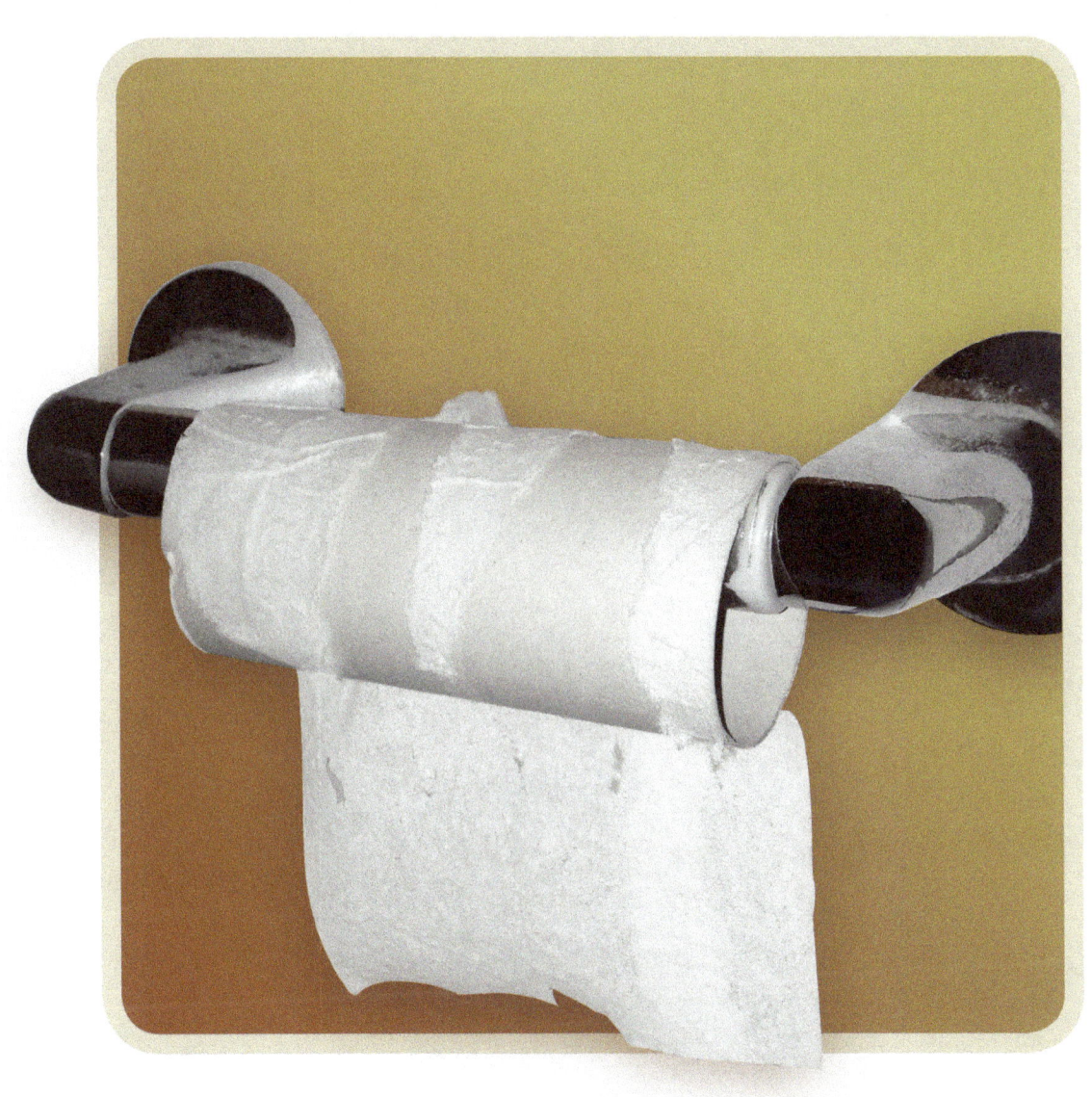

{ Of course I'm panicking.
Somebody has to. }

PANIC DISORDER

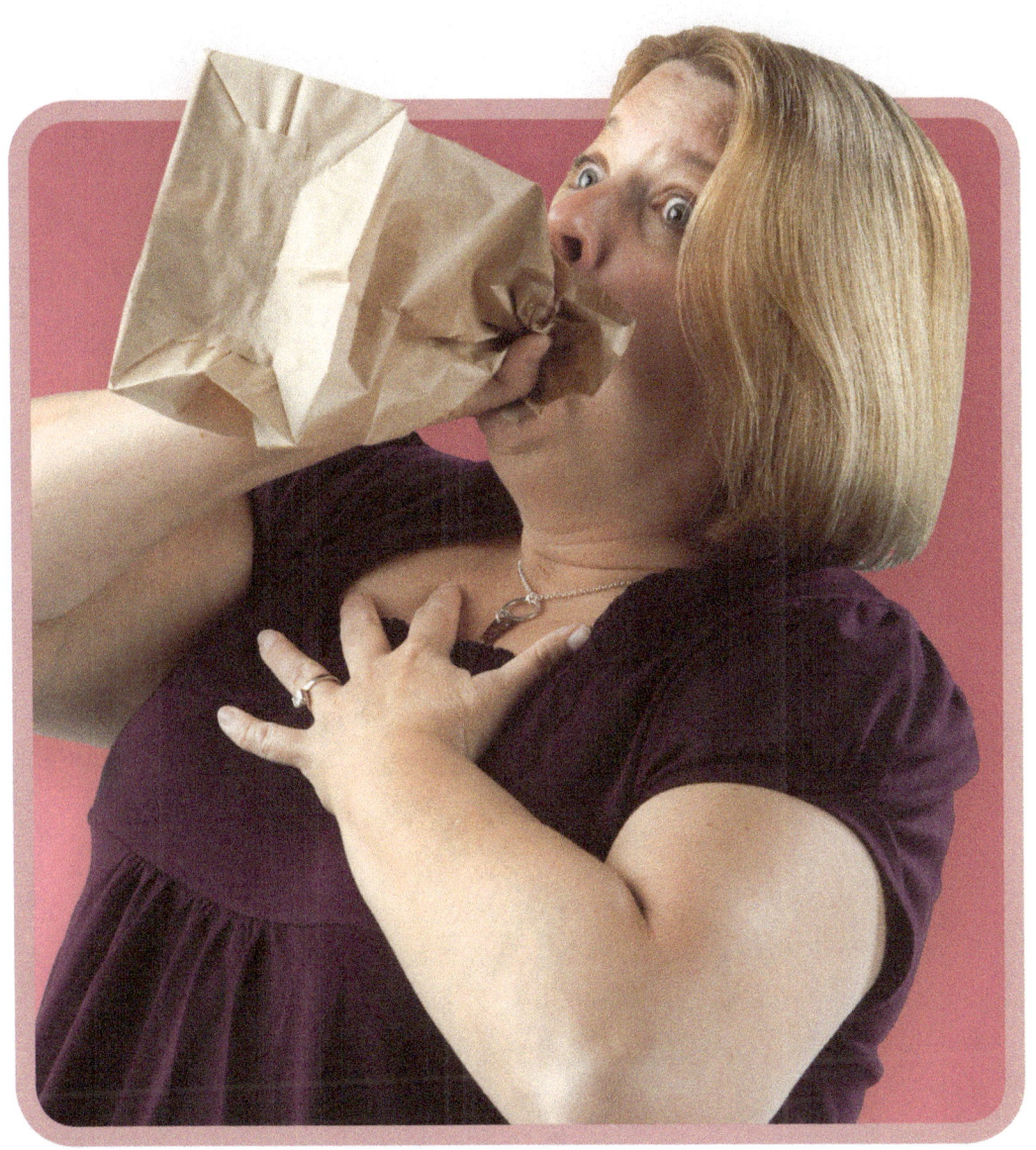

{ Careful—my tension level is @ Code Red. }

ANXIETY

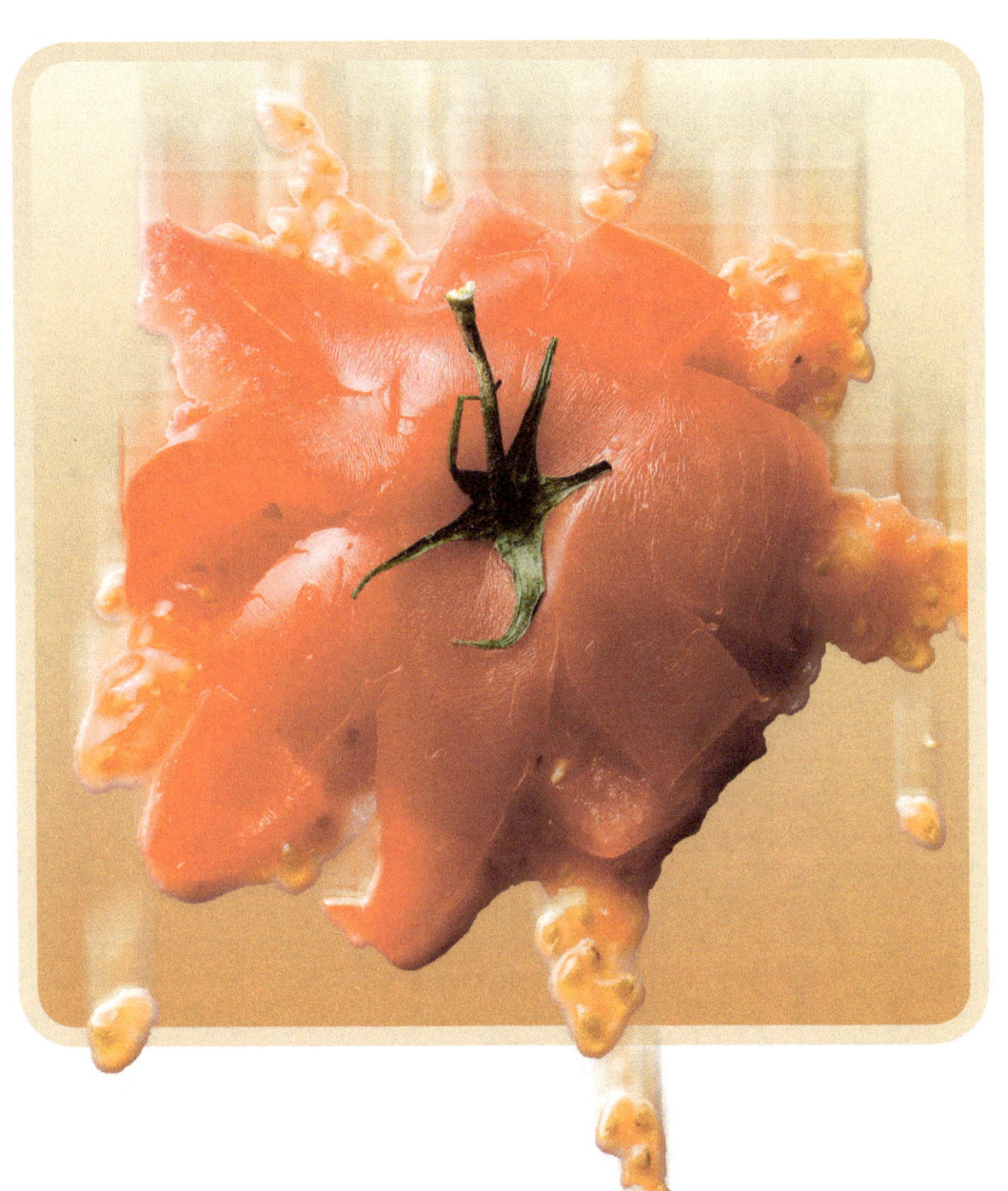

{ I'm becoming
allergic to everything.
When ice cream
makes that list, shoot me. }

ALLERGIES

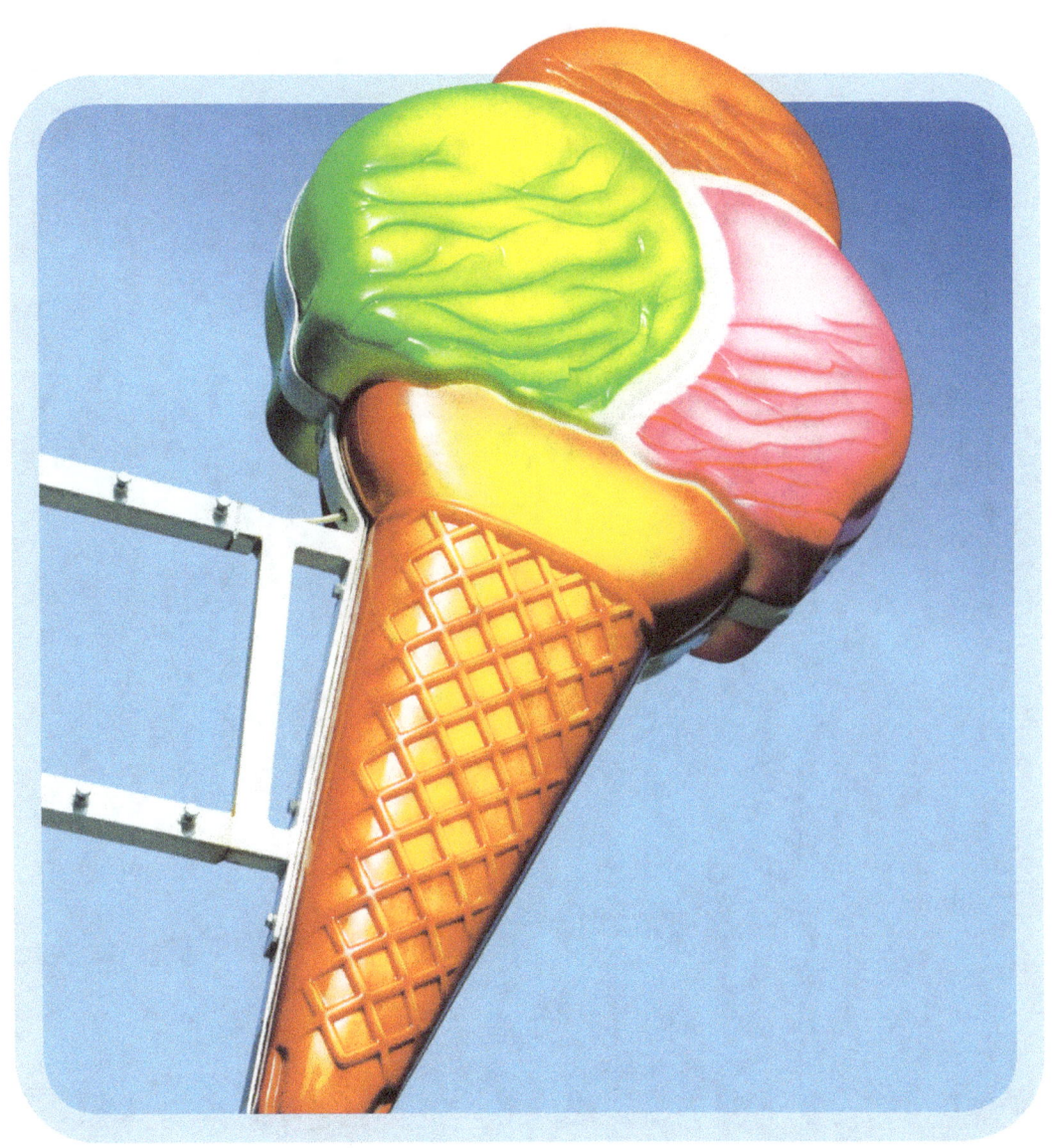

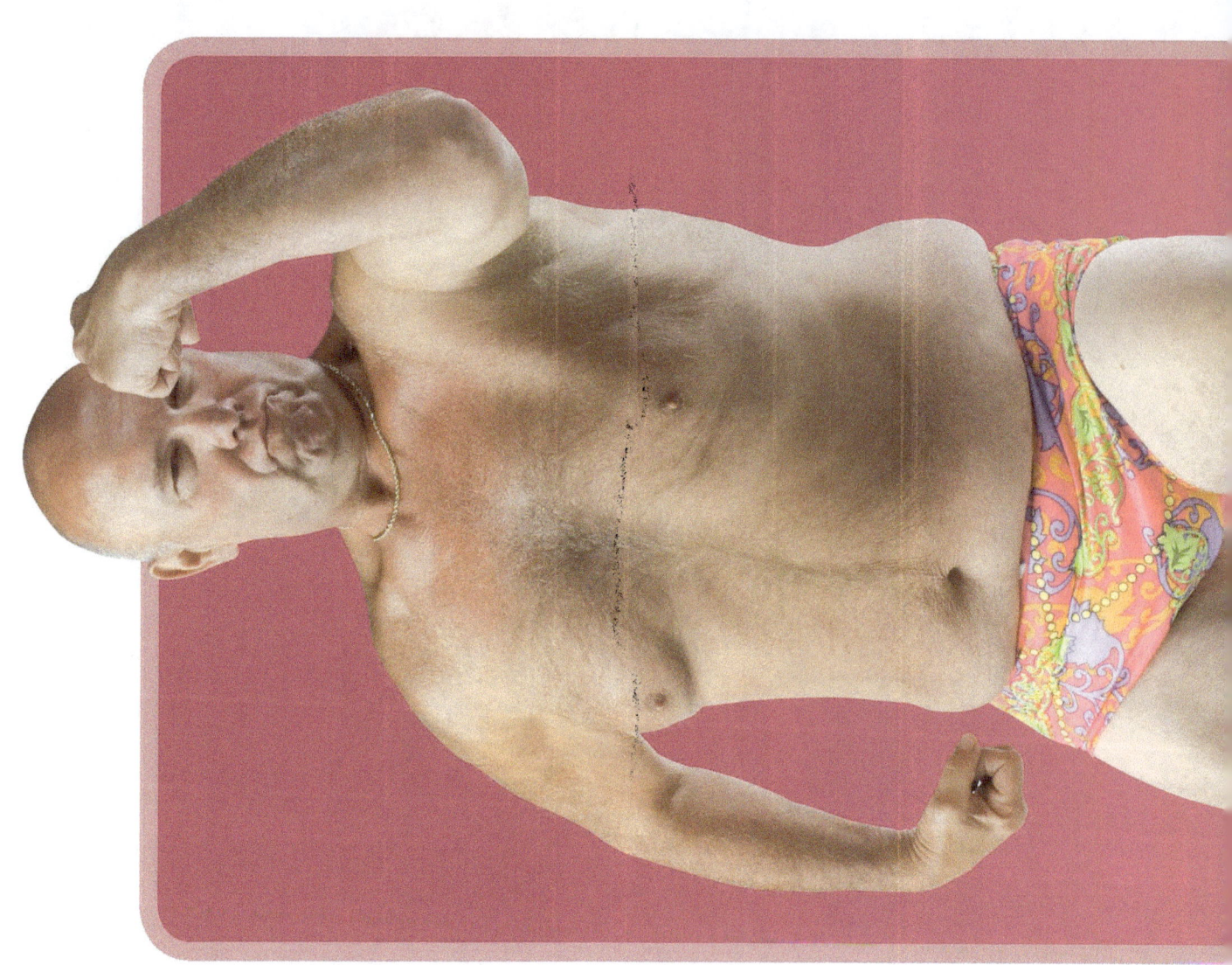

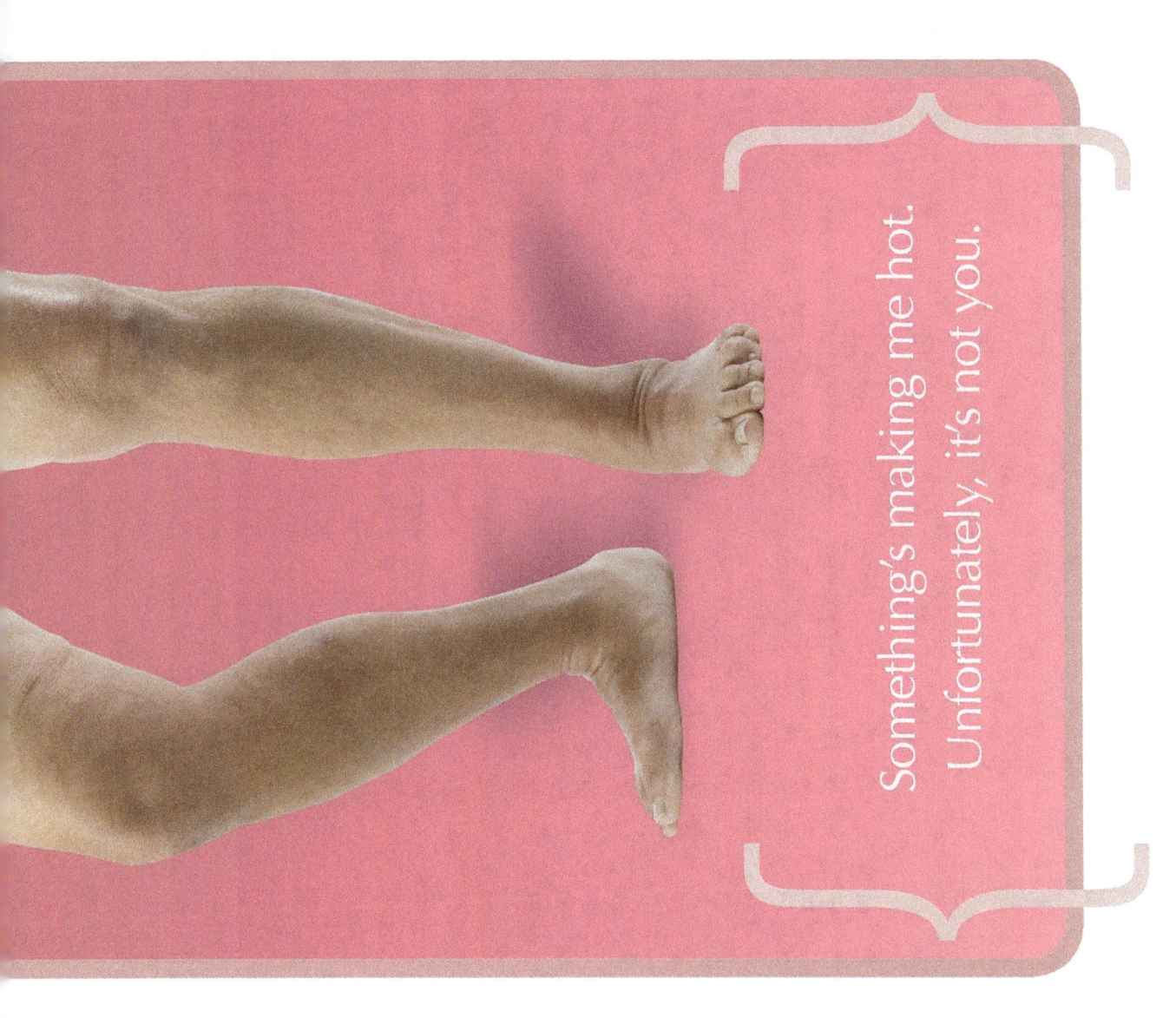

{ For now, consider sex a DIY project. }

LIBIDO LA BYE-BYE

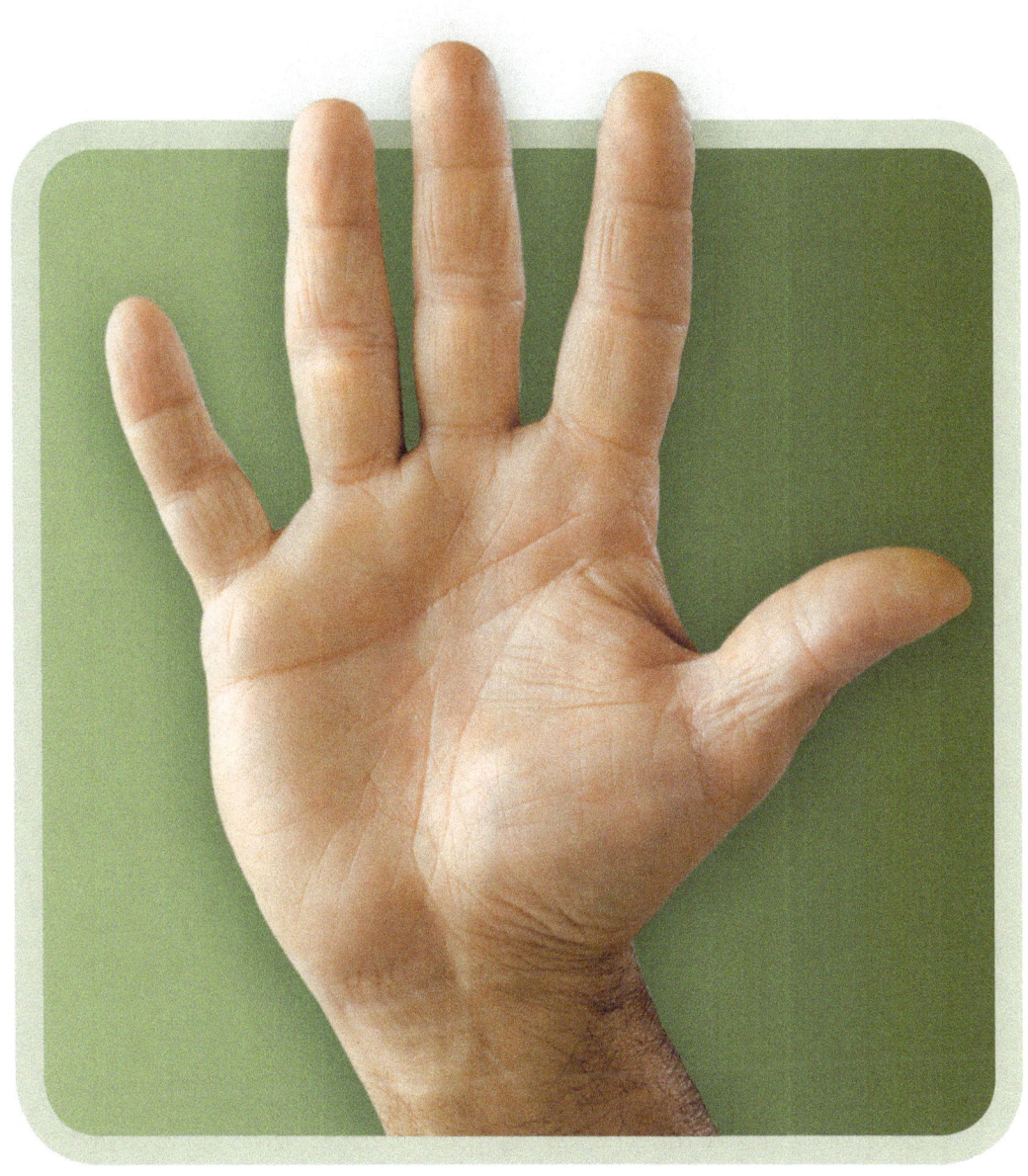

{ How can
the front of my neck
be so saggy when the back
is tighter than our
grocery budget? }

MUSCLE TENSION

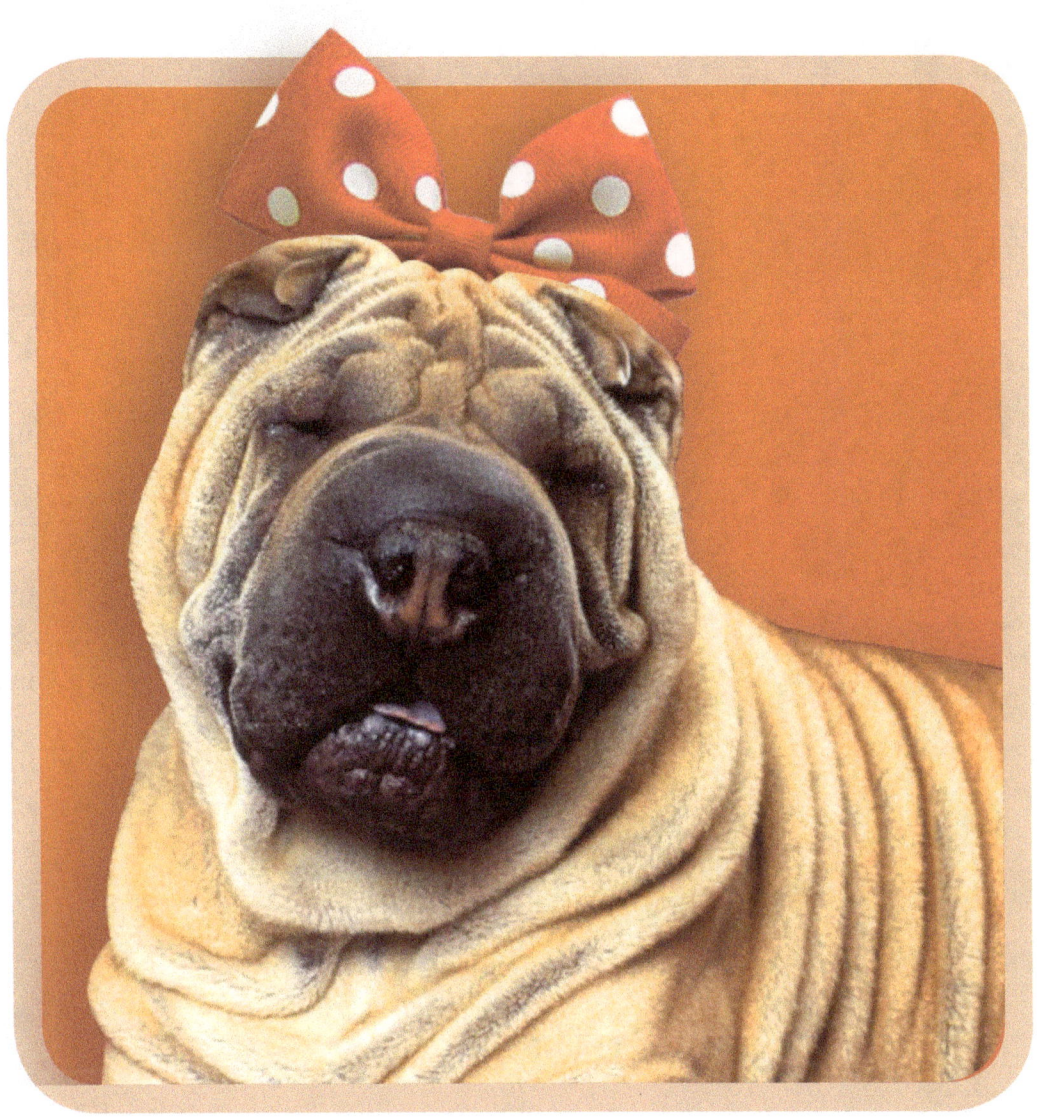

{ Everytime I sneeze,
I blow out a panty liner. }

INCONTINENCE

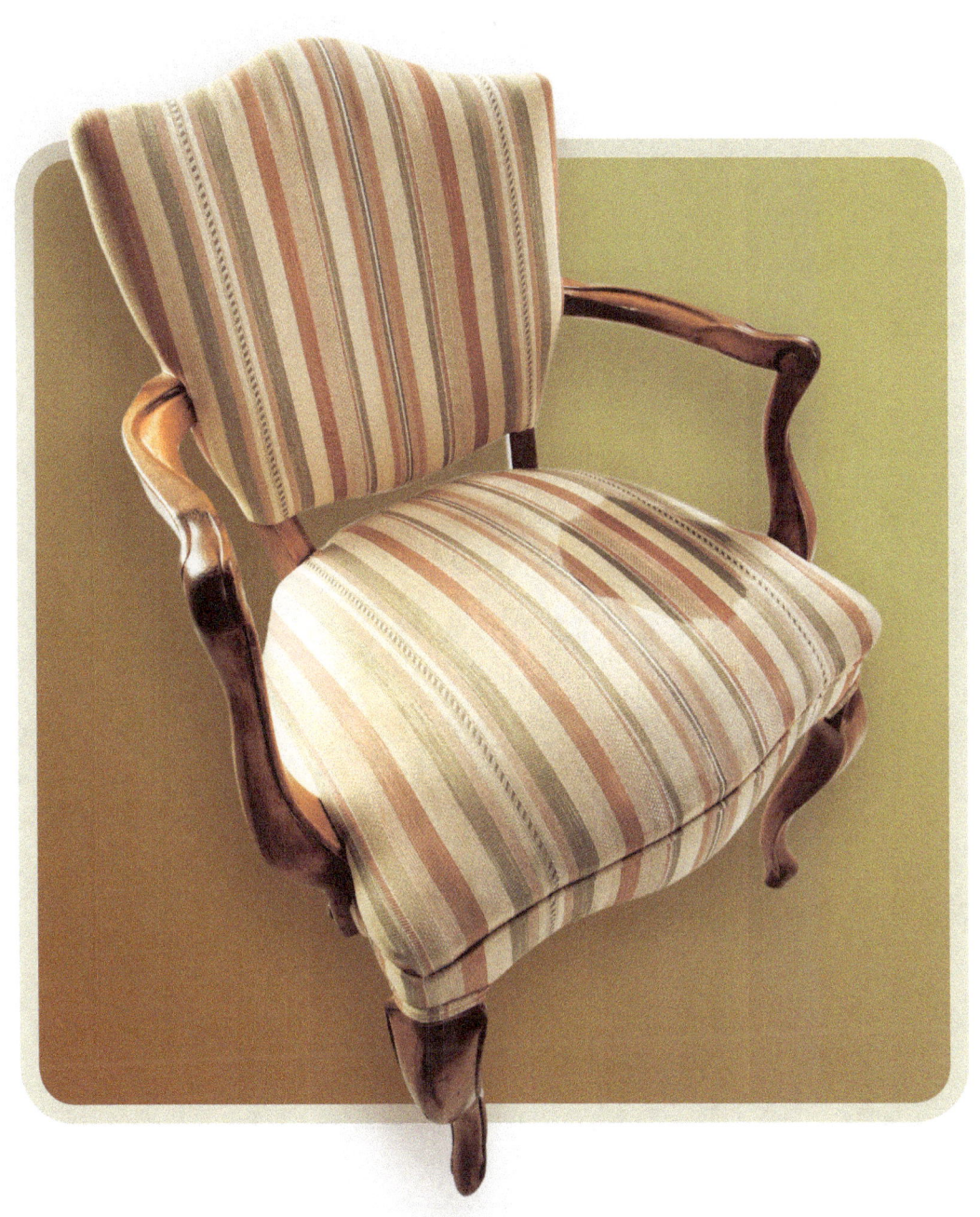

{ Trust me.
My morning stiffness
is *waaaaay* different
than yours. }

JOINT PAIN

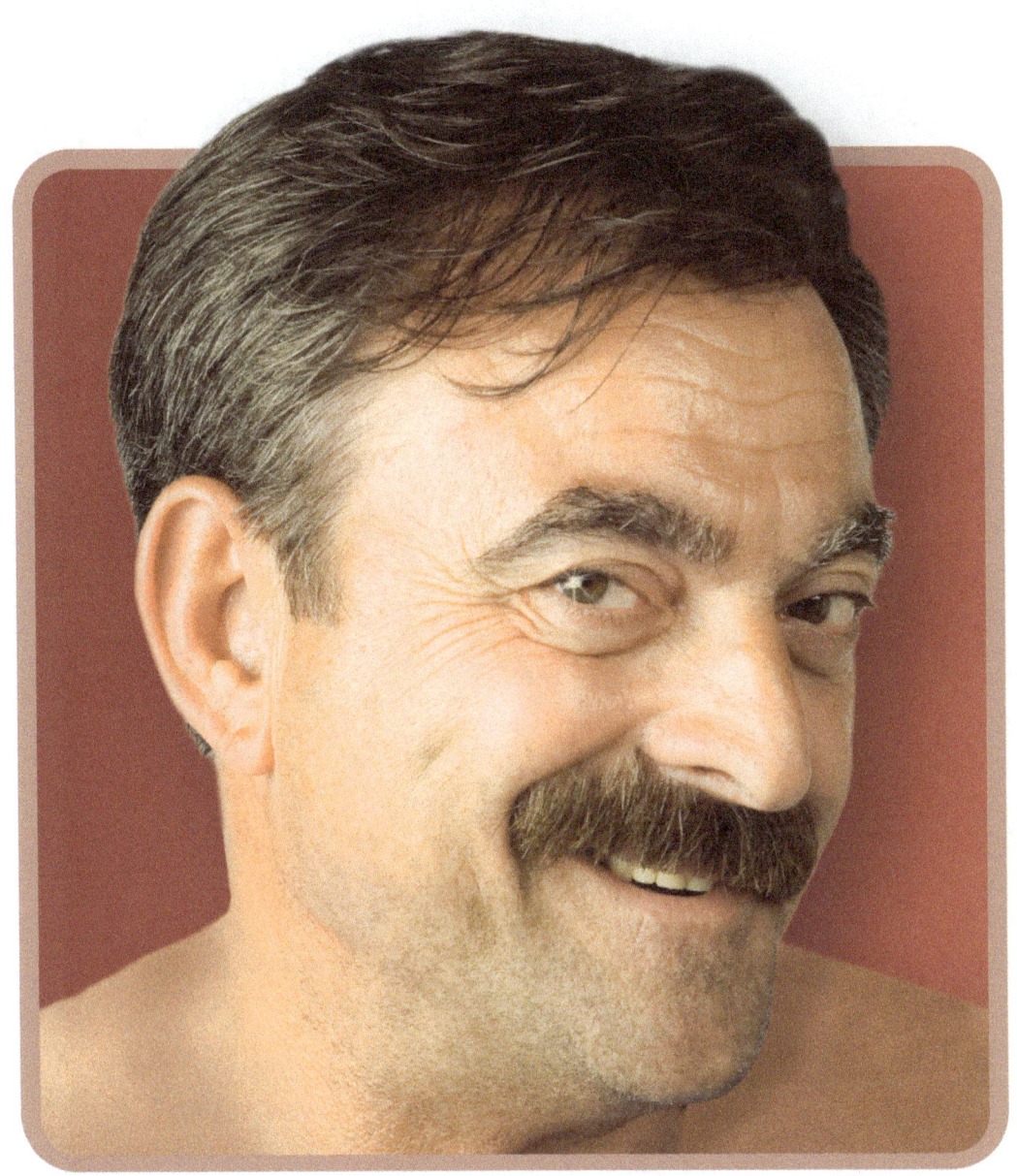

{ At least this time around, my pimples won't be immortalized in a yearbook. }

ADULT ACNE

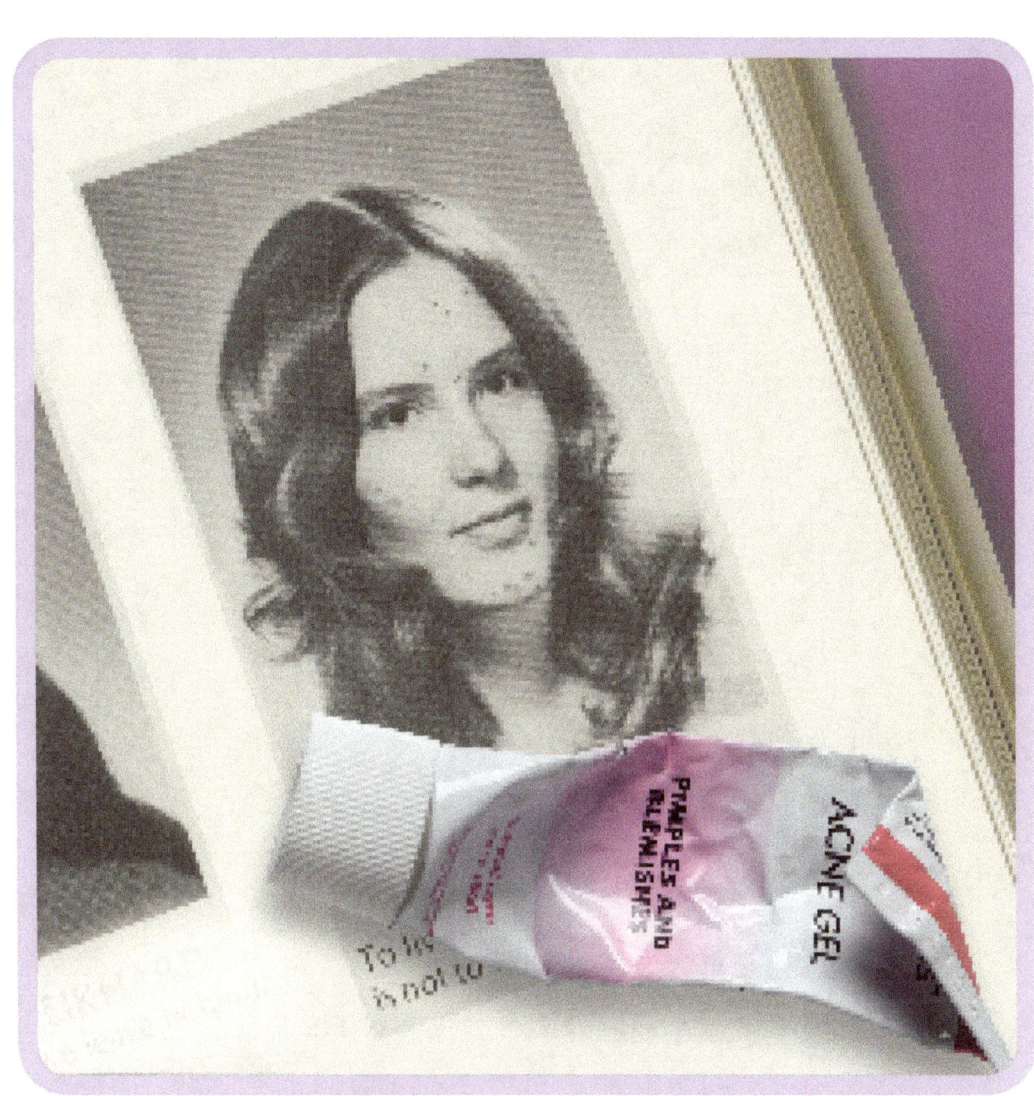

{ My boobs are so sensitive, they could read Braille. }

BREAST TENDERNESS

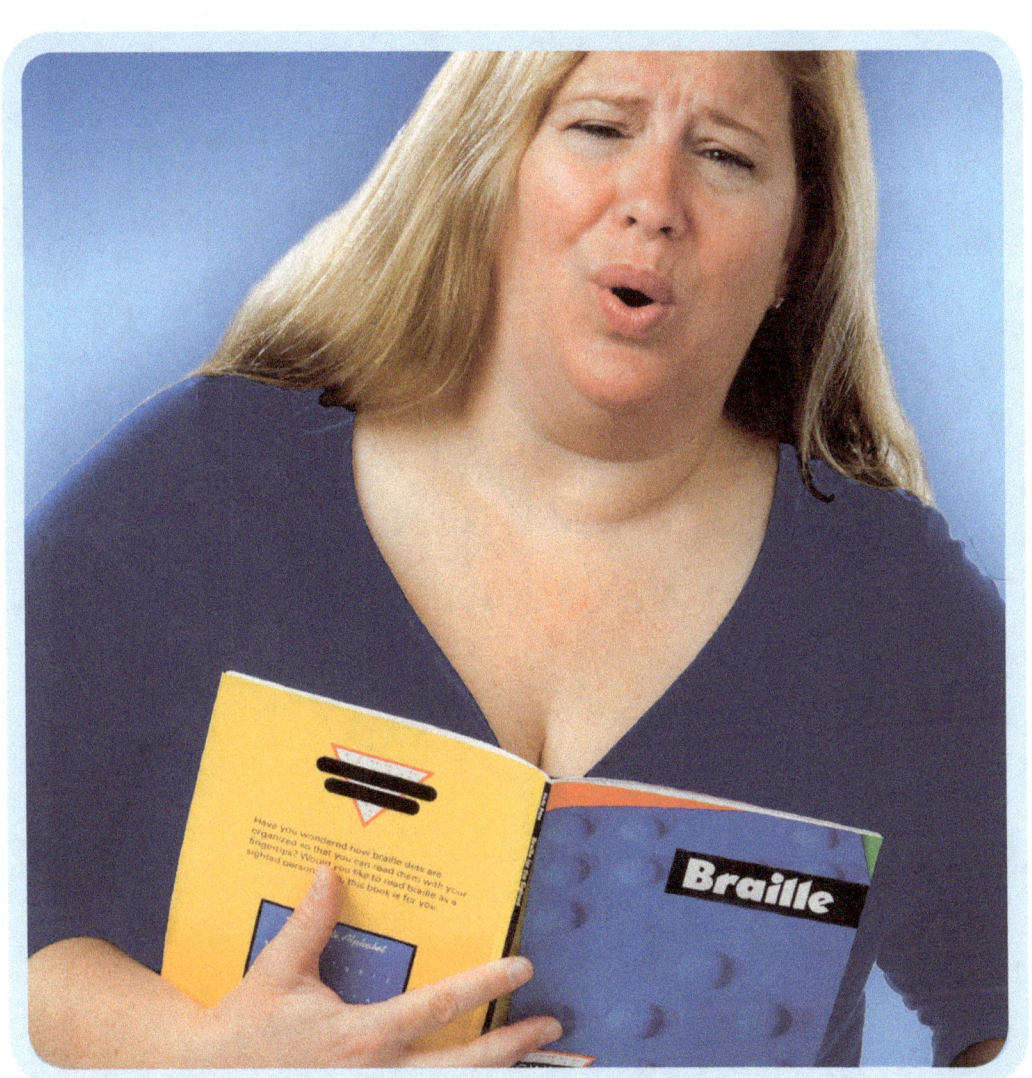

{ My heart used to race because my hormones were pumping. Now it races 'cause they're not. }

IRREGULAR HEARTBEAT

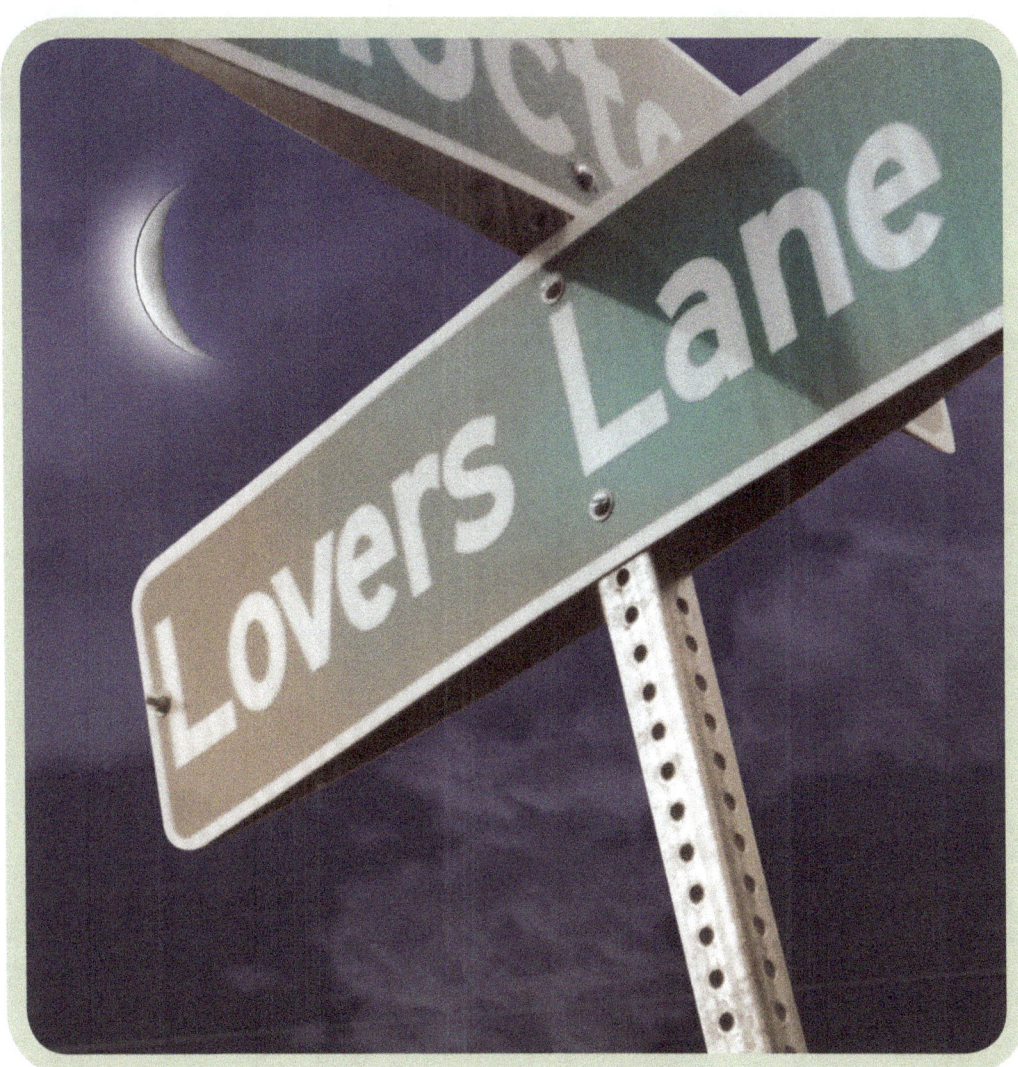

{ Some moisture problems can be solved with beer. Mine isn't one of them. }

VAGINAL DRYNESS

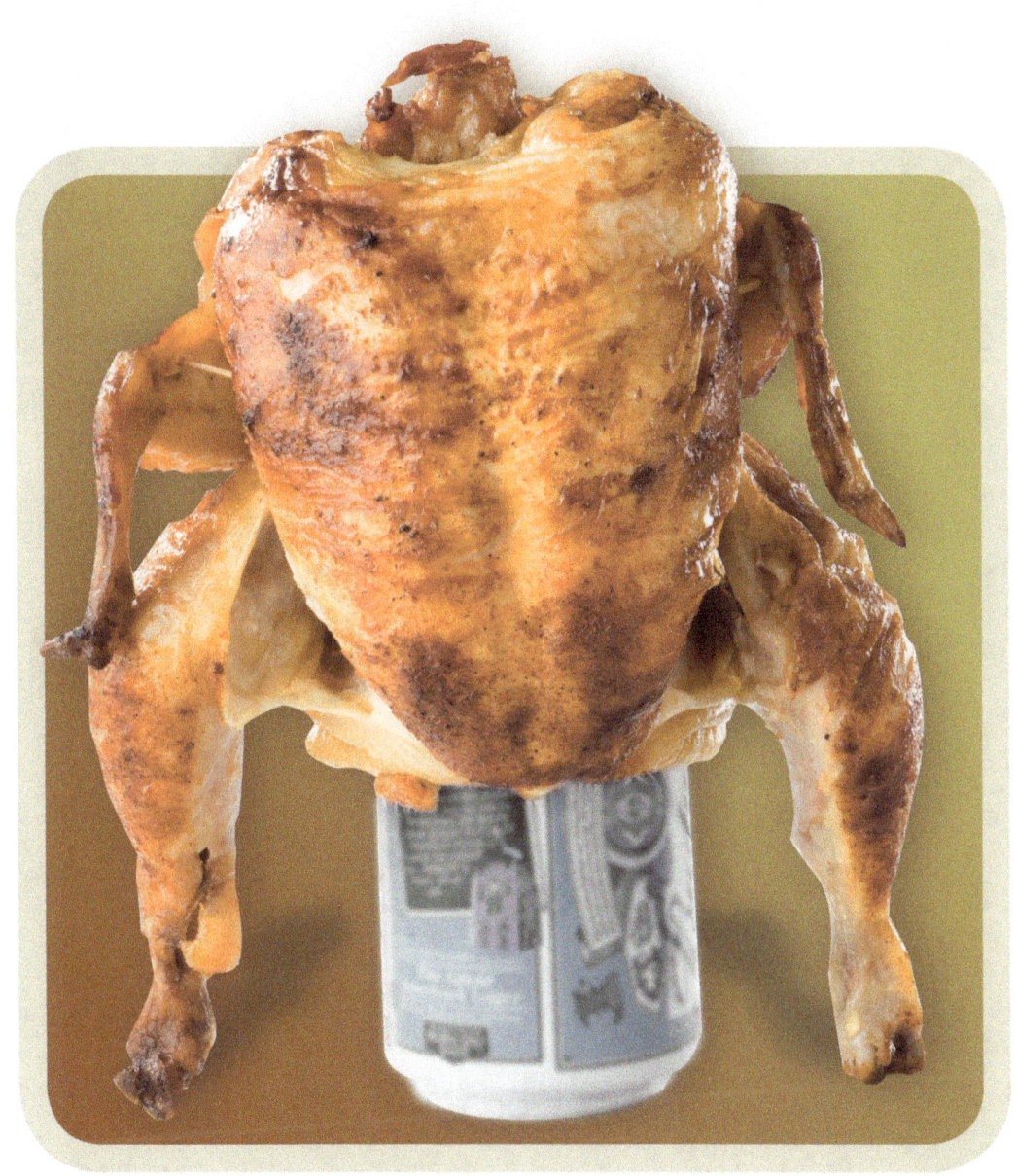

{ Horizontal is the new vertical. }

FATIGUE

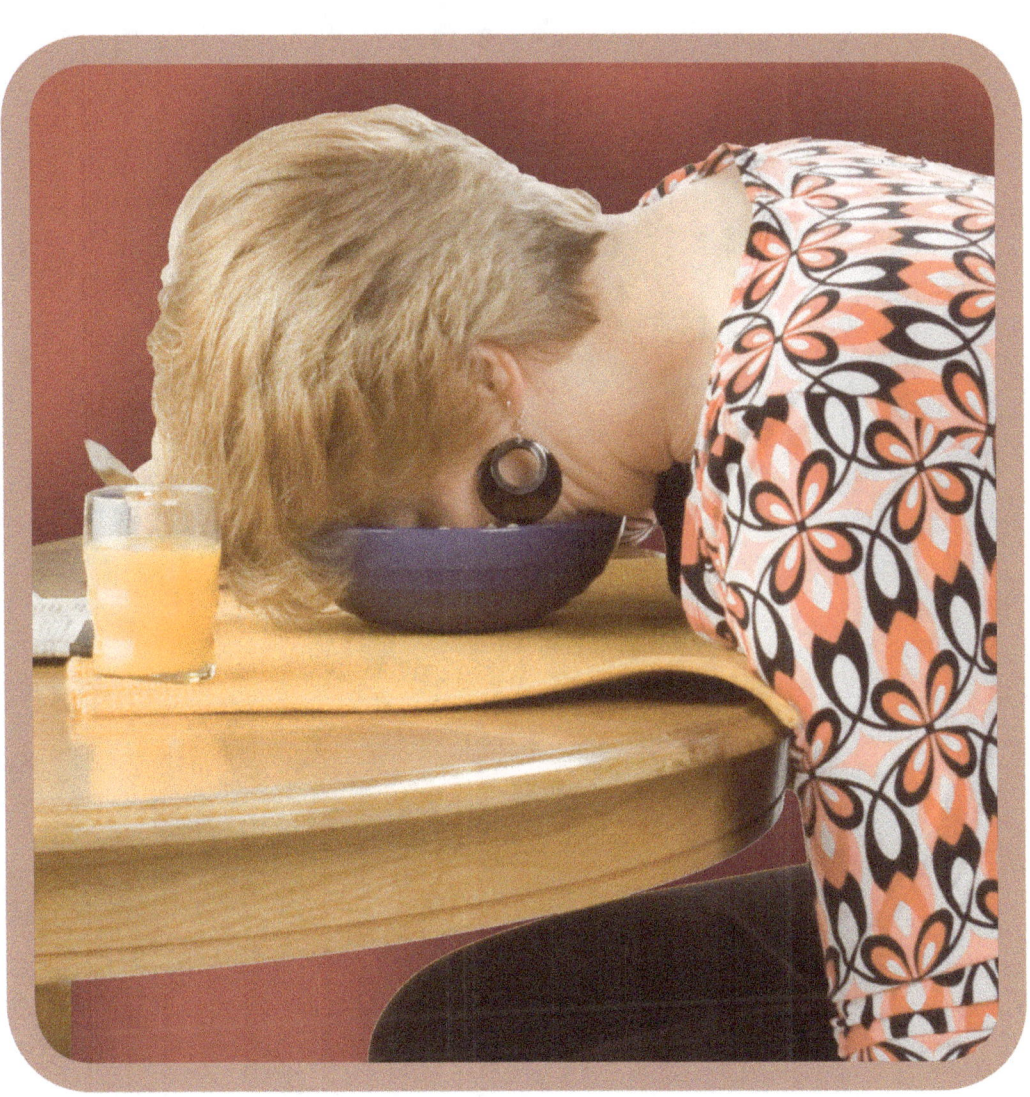

{ It's beyond manicure.
I need a menocure. }

BRITTLE NAILS

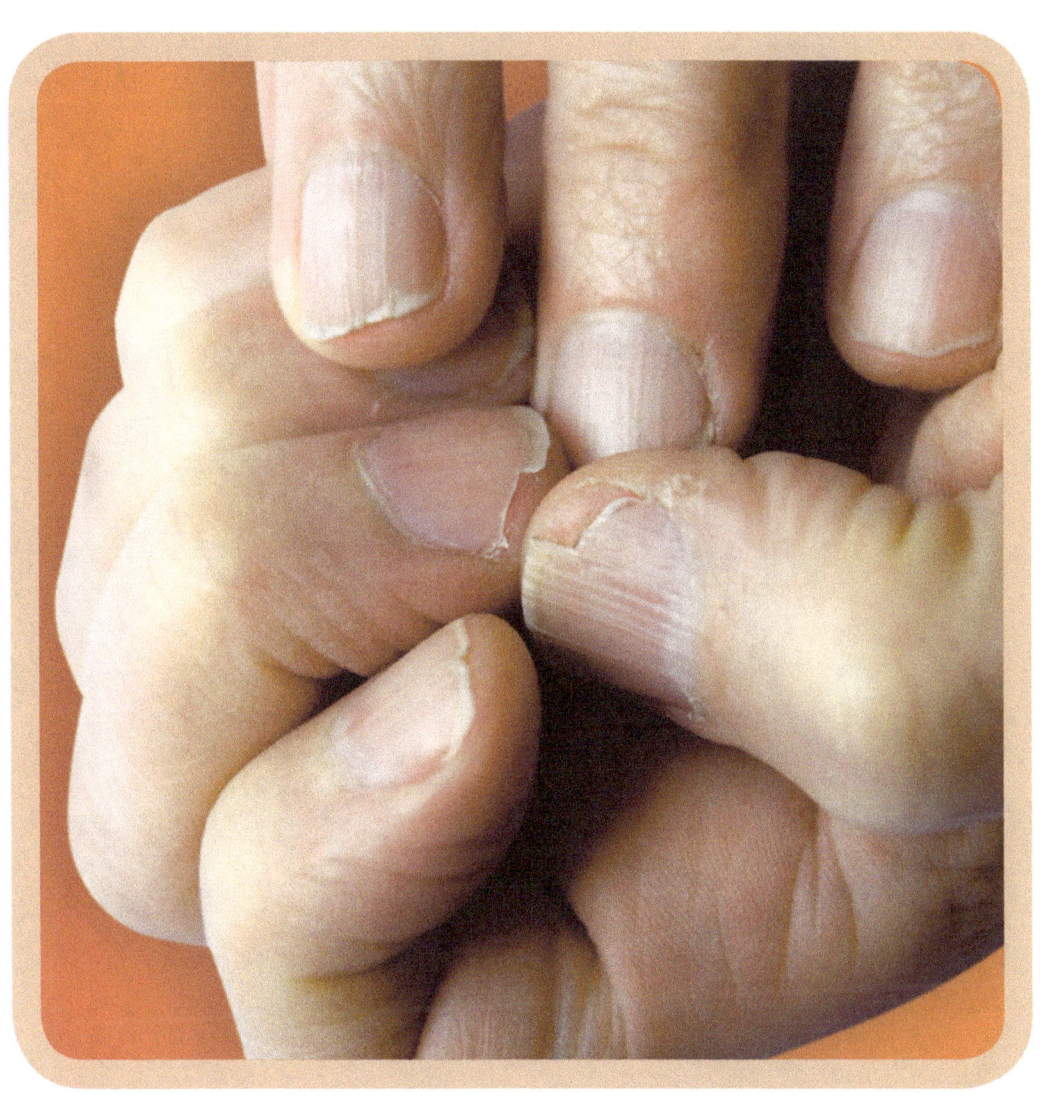

{ No,
my evening primrose,
black cohash
and St. John's wort
aren't part of the Dark Arts. }

HERBAL REMEDIES

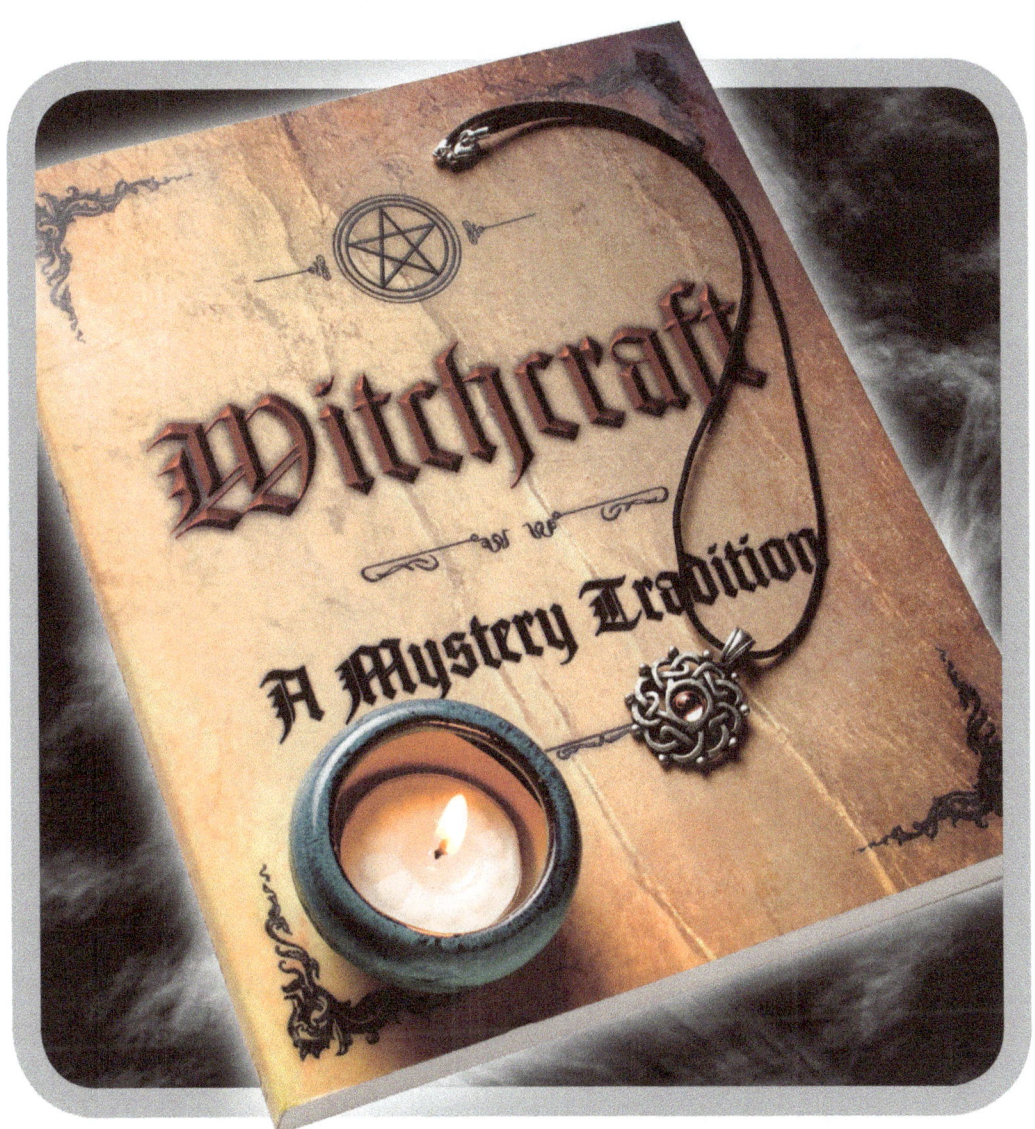

{ The 7-year itch?
Ha!
Try the 24/7 itch. }

ITCHY SKIN

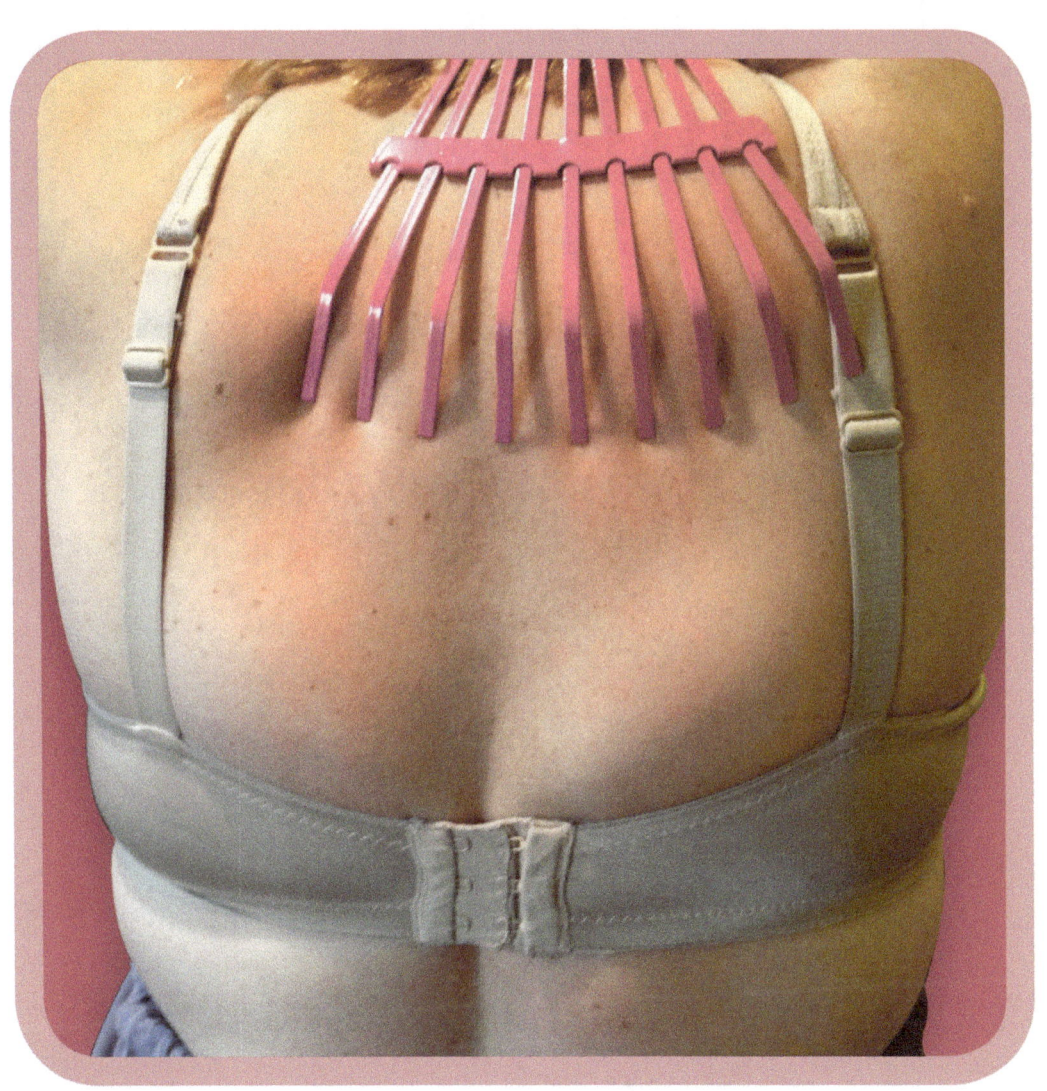

{ I can't sleep,
but at least I'm recycling. }

SLEEP DISORDERS

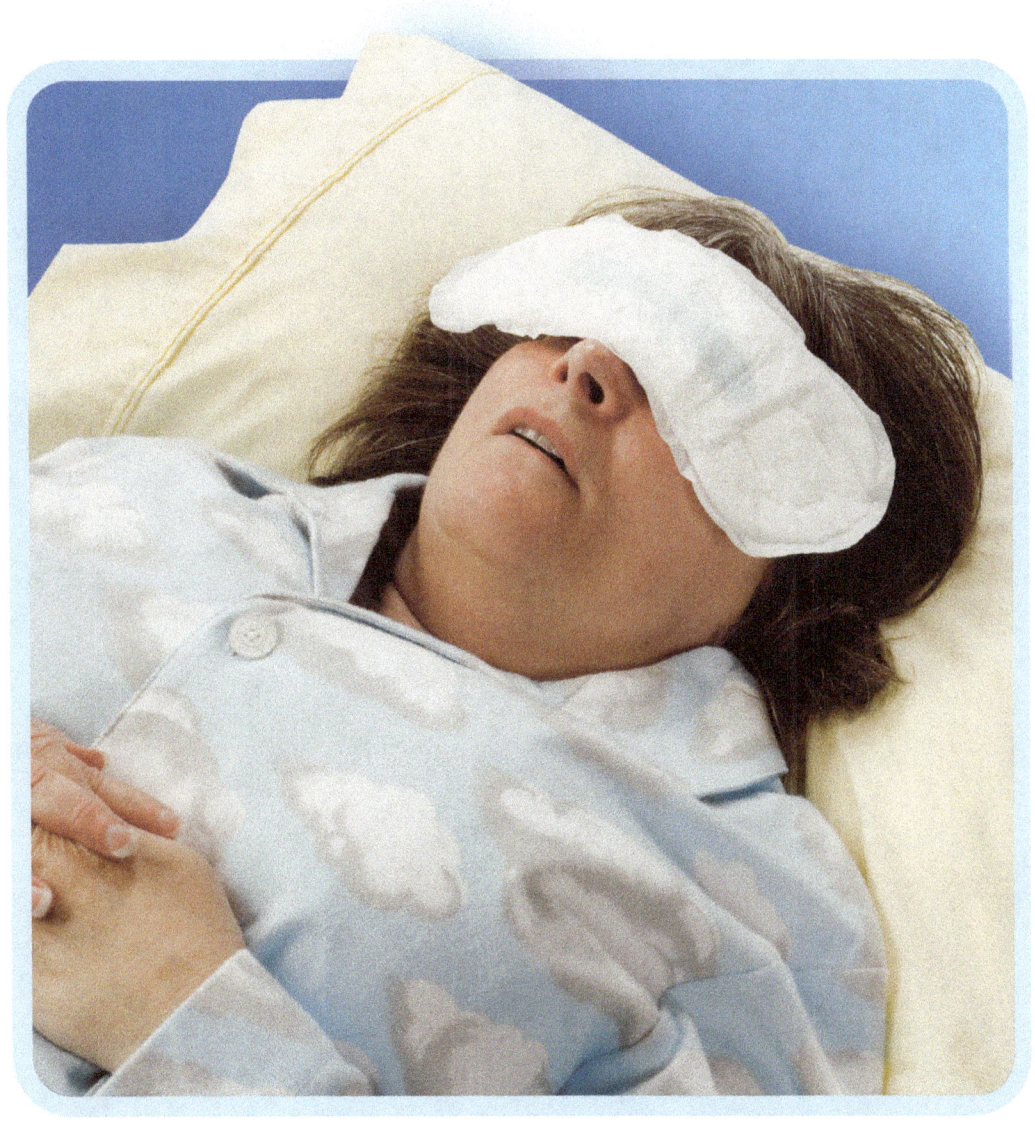

{ My fantasizing
about your death…
doesn't mean
I don't love you. }

IRRITABILITY

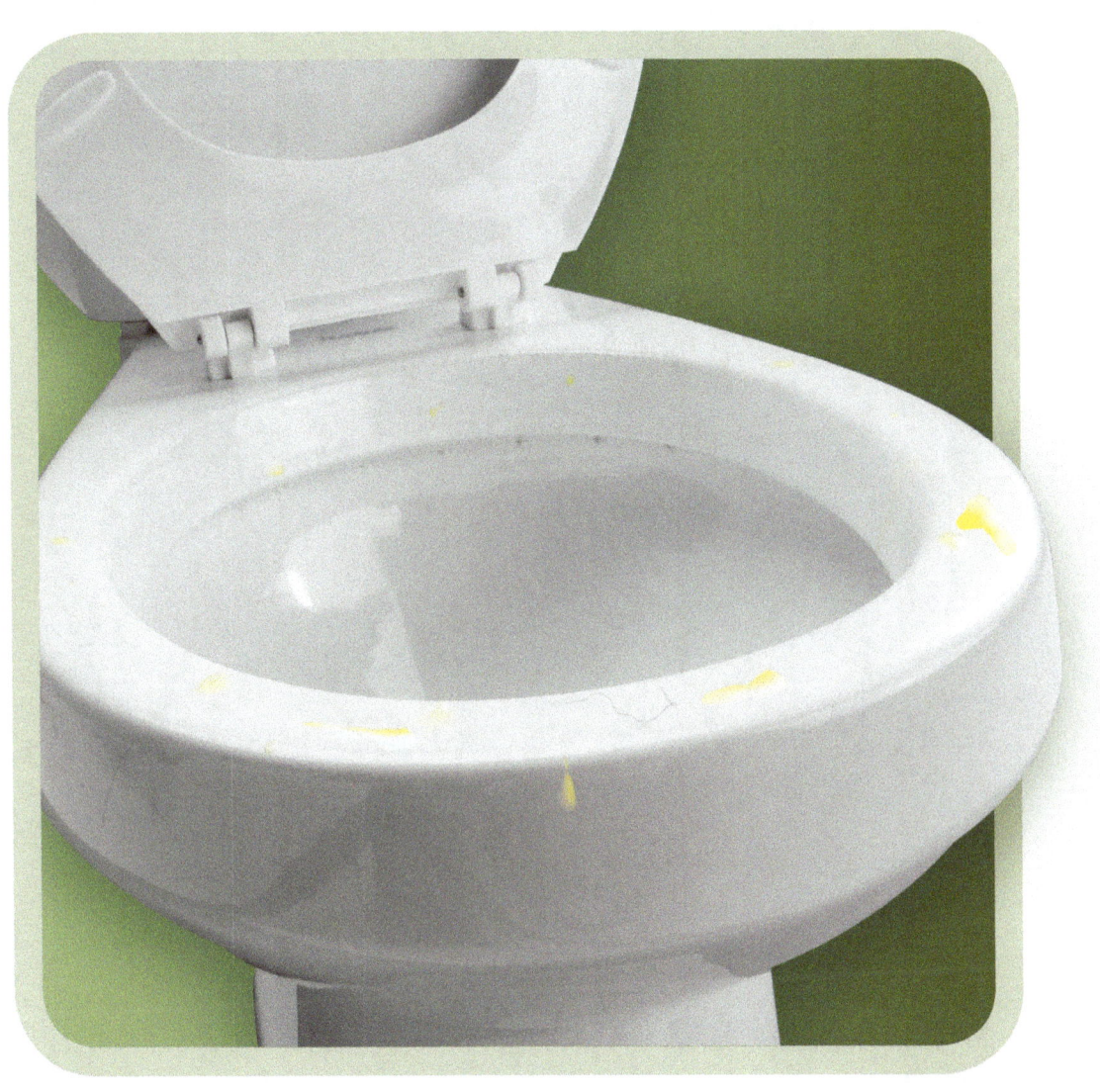

{ My bones are so porous, my x-rays look like Swiss cheese. }

OSTEOPOROSIS

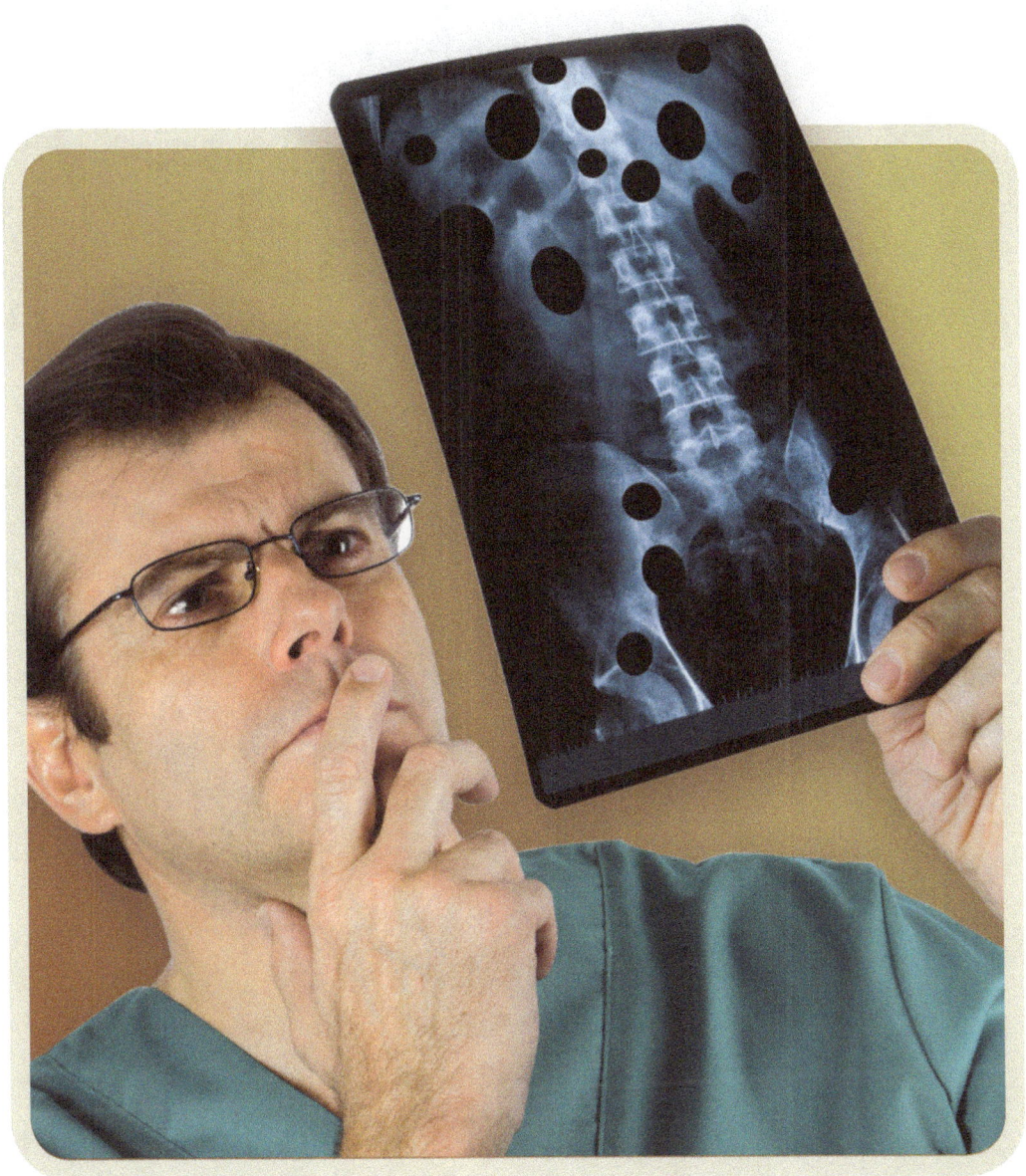

{ My period didn't
exactly stop —
it moved to my gums. }

BLEEDING GUMS

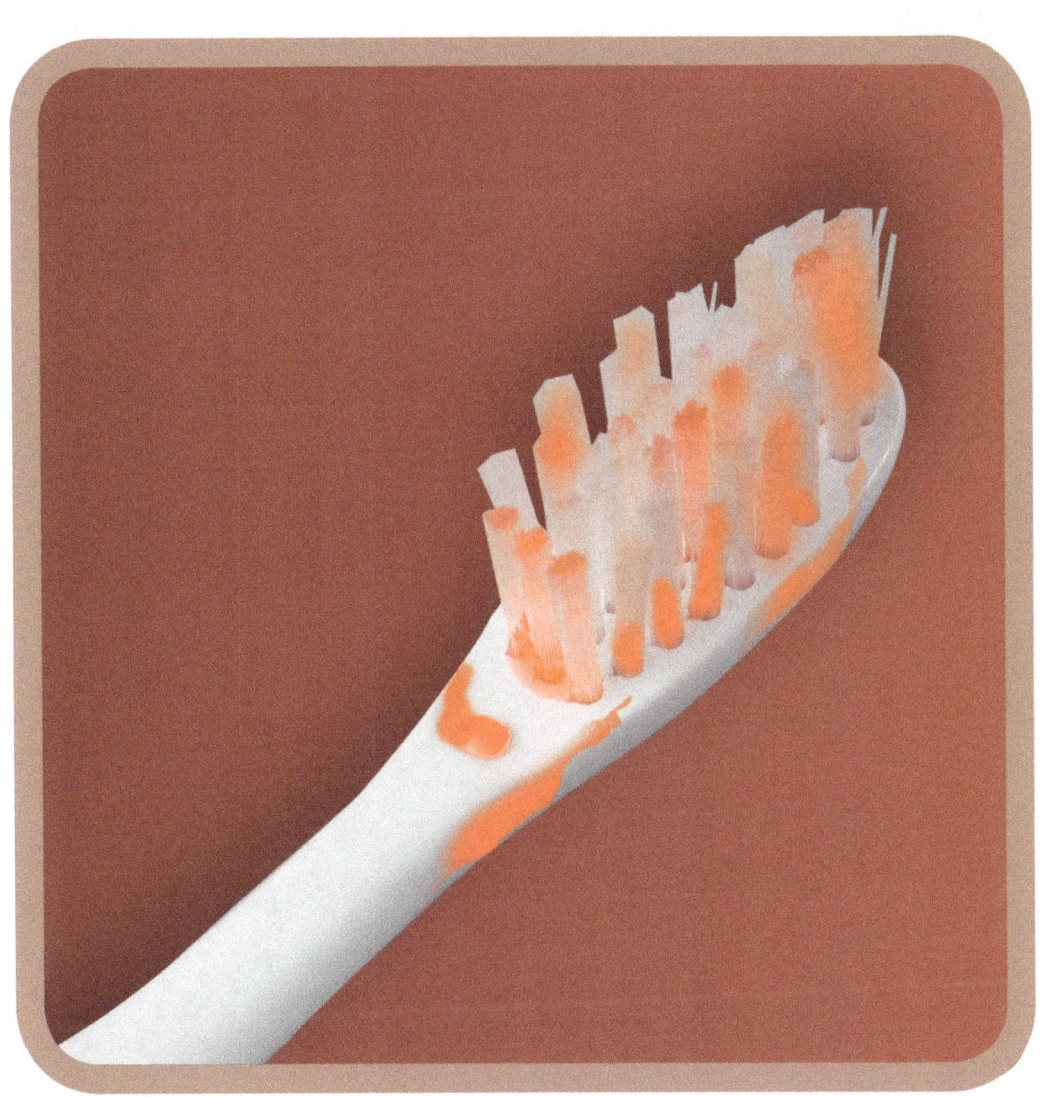

{ Thith ith how mah tuhng feelth. }

BURNING TONGUE

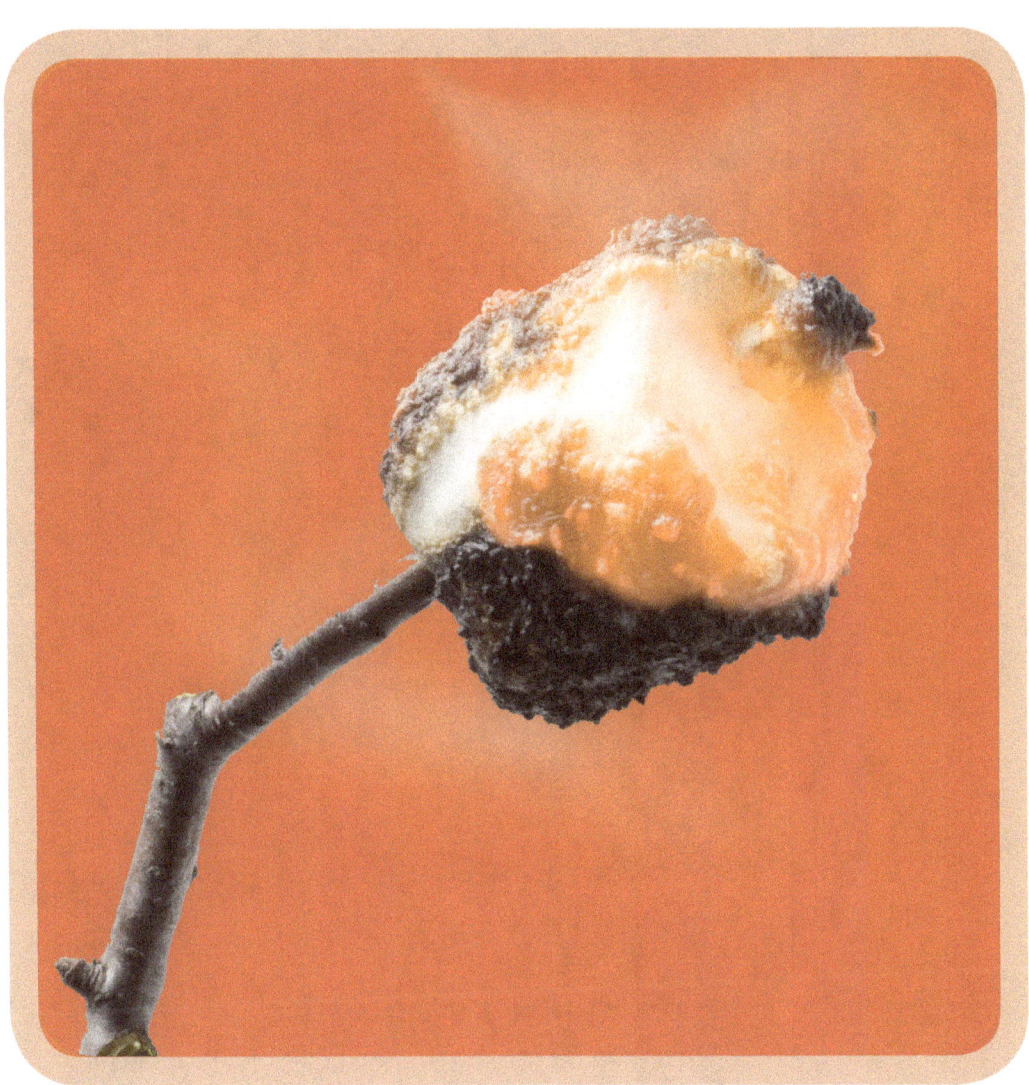

{ I don't care
how big you think
your generator is,
it won't jump-start
my libido. }

AWOL LIBIDO

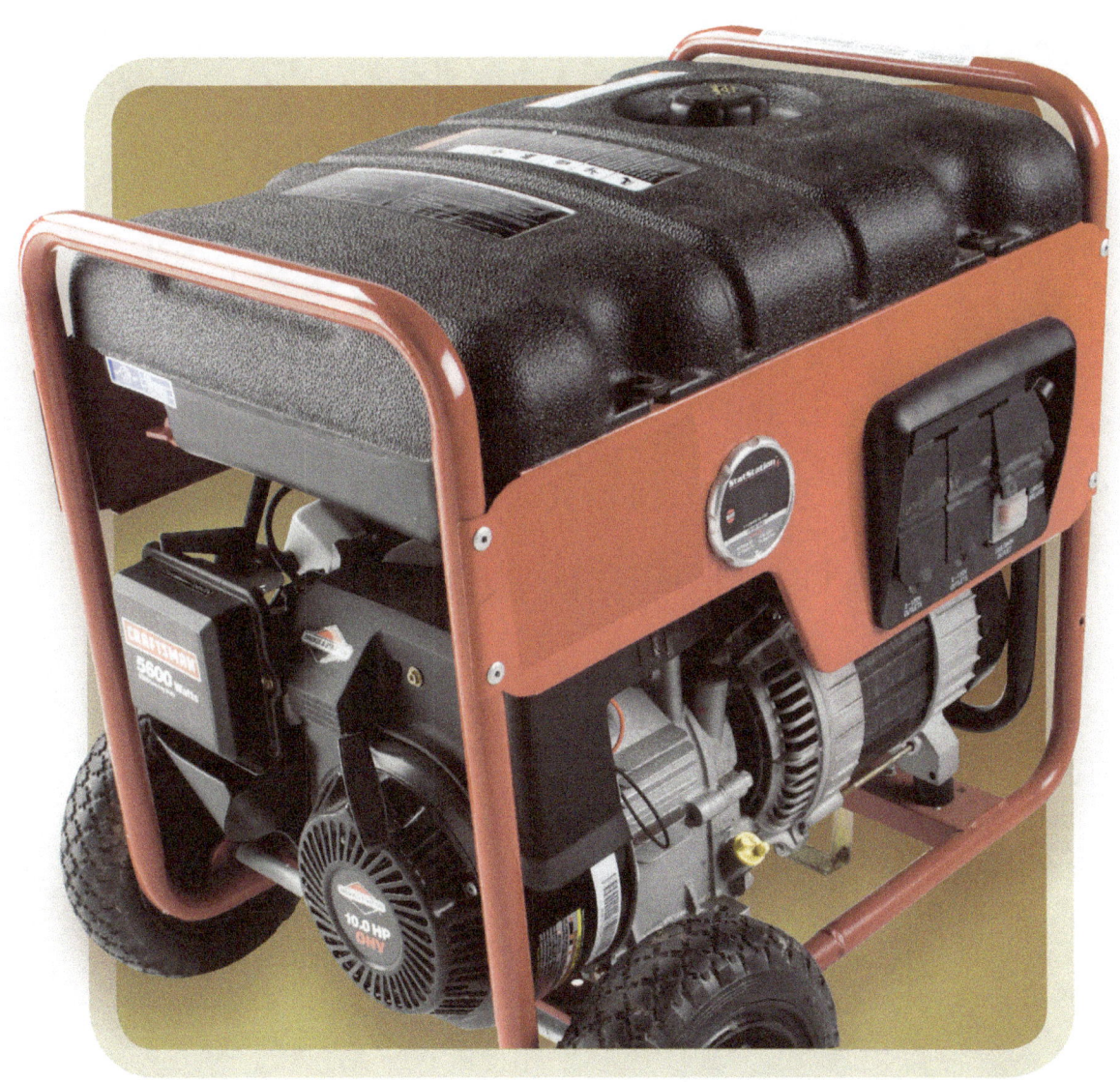

{ Sometimes
the room is spinning
so much, it appears
you're actually moving. }

DIZZINESS

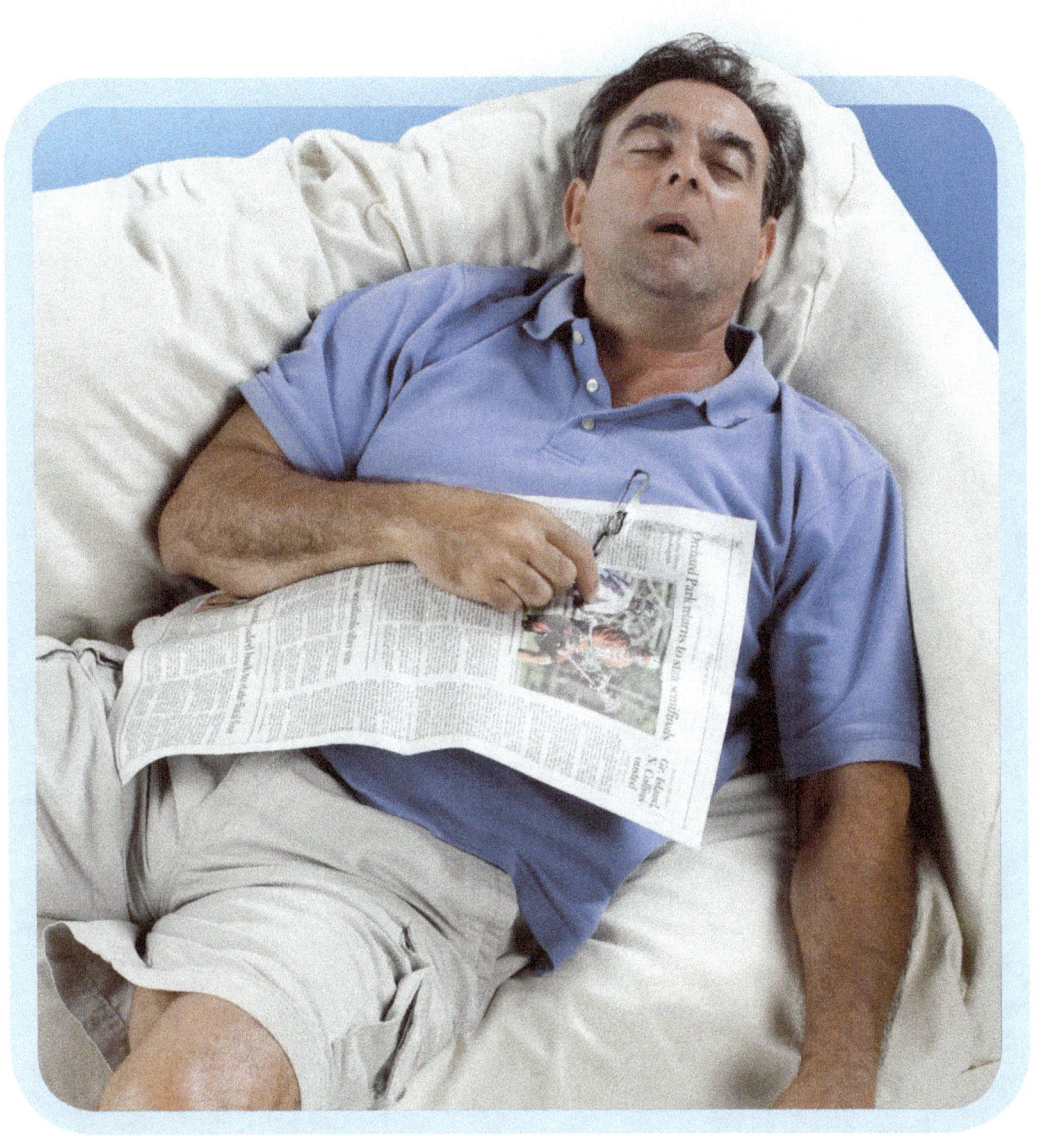

{ My deodorant may be strong enough for a man, but it's no match for menopause. }

ODOR CHANGES

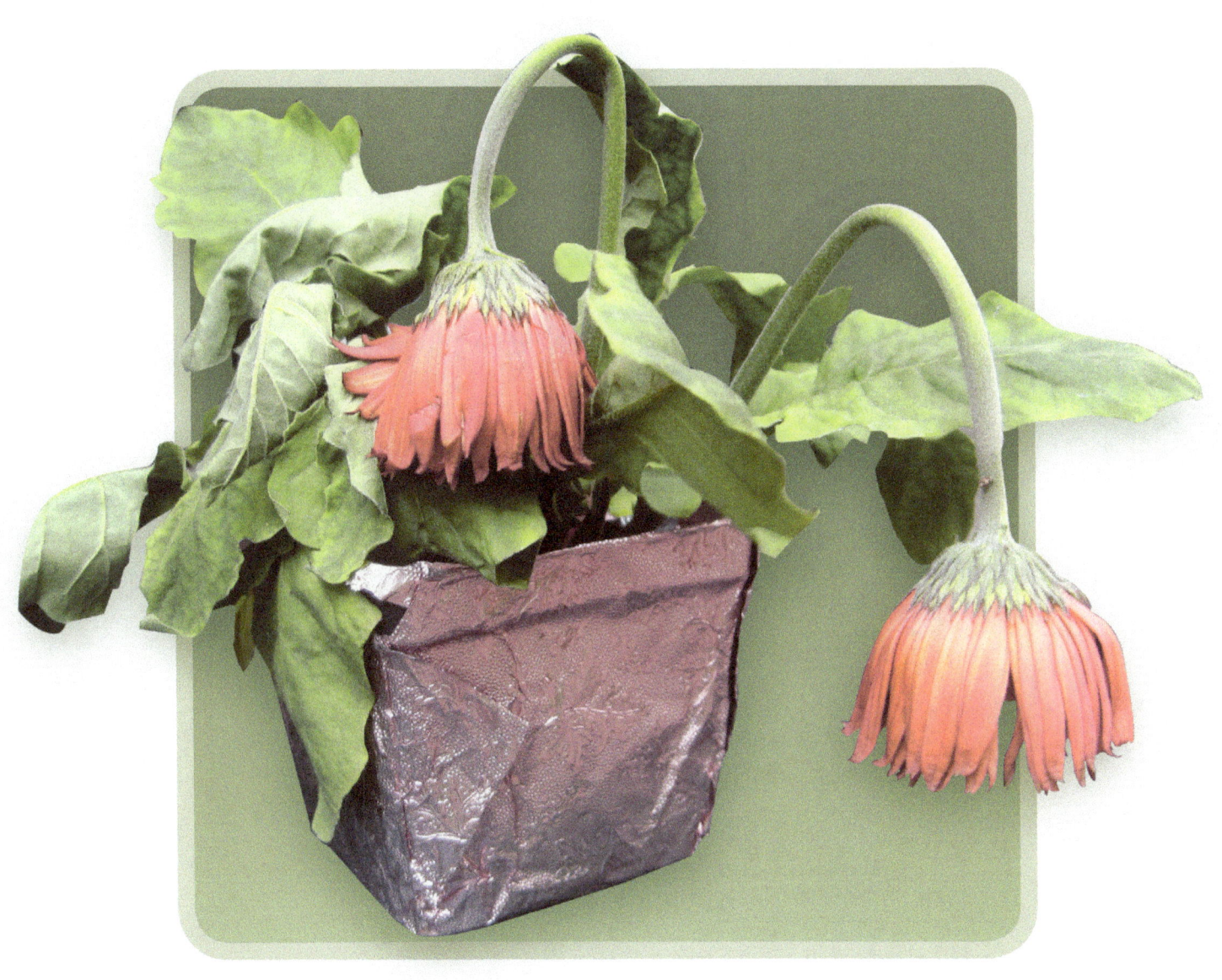

{ I laugh 'til I cry.
Except I leave out
the laughing part. }

DEPRESSION

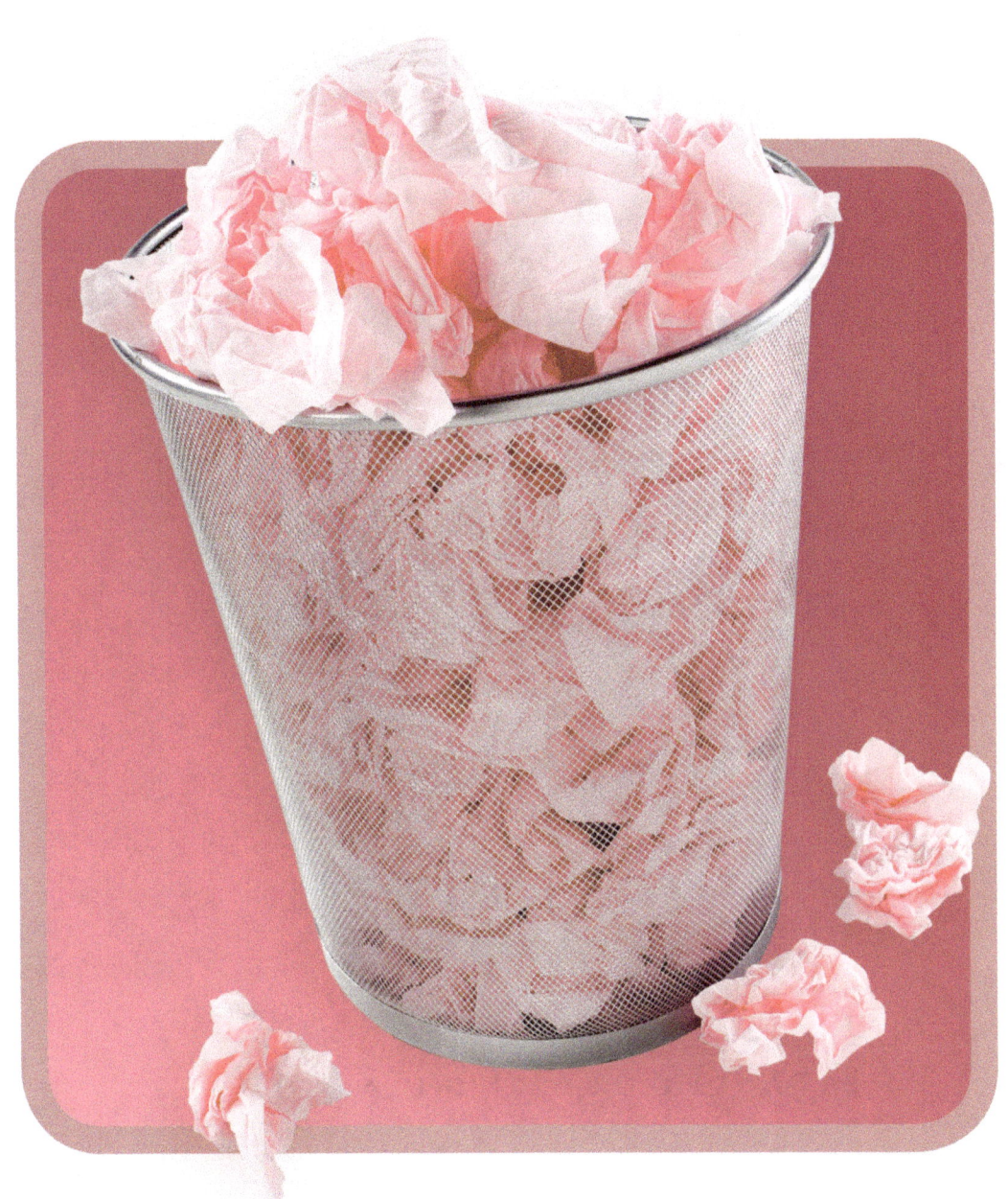

{ Gentlemen,
be nice and maybe
she'll let you live. }

BE A SPOUSE, NOT A LOUSE.

Help your partner survive the physical and mental trials of menopause. Be supportive, respond with compassion, and know when to get out of the way.

These suggestions will get you started in the right direction:

- Have her see a doctor to ensure her symptoms aren't something more serious.
- Give her back or foot rubs when she's achy.
- Help with household chores so she can get more rest.
- Take her out to a nice, relaxing dinner now and then.
- Don't make sexual demands when she's not in the mood.
- Dress in layers to accommodate her fluctuating temperature needs.
- Tell her you love her. Show her you love her.

"The Change" is different for every woman, but the effects will eventually end…in a year or ten. Be a supportive partner and your relationship will likely emerge stronger and more fulfilling in the post-menopausal years. Remember, your caring response to her needs now could have a positive impact on how diligently she changes your diapers when you reach senility.

www.ingramcontent.com/pod-product-compliance
Lightning Source LLC
Chambersburg PA
CBHW082245300426
44110CB00036B/2447